Telehealth in Urology

Telehealth in Urology

Dara Lundon

Department of Urology, Icahn School of Medicine at Mount Sinai Hospitals, New York, NY, USA

ELSEVIER

Telehealth in Urology   ISBN: 978-0-323-87480-9

Notices

Practitioners and researchers must always rely on their own experience and knowledge in evaluating and using any information, methods, compounds or experiments described herein. Because of rapid advances in the medical sciences, in particular, independent verification of diagnoses and drug dosages should be made. To the fullest extent of the law, no responsibility is assumed by Elsevier, authors, editors or contributors for any injury and/or damage to persons or property as a matter of products liability, negligence or otherwise, or from any use or operation of any methods, products, instructions, or ideas contained in the material herein.

Publisher: Dolores Meloni
Acquisitions Editor: Belinda Kuhn
Editorial Project Manager: Billie Jean Fernandez
Project Manager: Kiruthika Govindaraju
Cover Designer: Greg Harris

3251 Riverport Lane
St. Louis, Missouri 63043

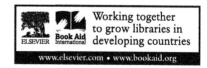

Contents

PART 2 How do I get started providing a telehealth service?

PART 3 What telehealth tools are available for urology?

Regulations concerning telehealth provision

Regulations and requirements for telehealth provision

Introduction

At the time of writing, a unique set of circumstances exist in the United States and elsewhere whereby the barriers to practice telehealth are minimal. In fact, if a licensed urologist in the USA has a smart phone, they are sufficiently equipped, and in compliance with regulations, to provide clinical consults to their patients via telehealth. On January 31, 2020, the 2019 Novel Coronavirus (COVID-19) was declared a public health emergency in the United States and a raft of subsequent legislation was passed, which cease to have effect at some date in relation to the end of this public health emergency. In terms of telehealth provisions, probably the chief among these came on March 17, 2020, when the Office for Civil Rights at the United States Department of Health and Human Services (HHS) announced that it would waive potential penalties for violations of Health Insurance Portability and Accountability Act of 1996 (HIPAA) against healthcare providers that serve patients through everyday communication technologies during the COVID-19 nationwide public health emergency. Thus, in effect, opening the door for any and all applications to be used to deliver telehealth by providers. The press release specifically named communication applications FaceTime and Skype and specified they could be used for any telehealth treatment or diagnostic purpose. After this expires, in the United States at least, all providers will be required to comply with relevant legislation. It should be remembered though that these regulations are not mere bureaucratic barriers to be overcome and, particularly in the case of laws relating to patient data and privacy, they exist to protect the best interests of patients and the medical profession. Just because physicians will not be fined for knowingly sharing patient information in insufficiently secure communications, does not mean that physicians should be doing so.

Regulation of telehealth is currently relatively relaxed in most jurisdictions and there is no one regulator of telehealth. In the United States and European Union (EU), each state has regulatory institutions that establish and dictate the standards for clinical treatment: for the most part, these same bodies regulate telemedicine and telehealth standards. However, these standards are often vague, and poorly defined. And while these state-level bodies operate in accordance with federal

Telehealth in Urology. https://doi.org/10.1016/B978-0-323-87480-9.00009-9

regulations such as rules from the Centers for Medicare and Medicaid Services (CMS), as mentioned, the extent and scope of these regulations pertaining to telemedicine is limited.

As the majority of telehealth regulation is determined on a state-by-state level in the United States and EU, it will not be dealt with in detail in this book. However, the Federation of State Medical boards (FSMB), the American Medical Association (AMA), and the Center for Connected Health Policy offer state-by-state guidance. The federally funded Center for Connected Health Policy in the United States is a great resource for federal and state-by-state policies affecting telehealth practice in the United States of America.

Given these caveats, there are some key laws and regulations that address essential criteria, which must be fulfilled to legally provide telehealth services. Some of the key federal regulations in the United States include the HIPAA, the Medicare Telehealth Services Flexibility Act (MTSFA), and the Federal Communication Commission's (FCC's) Rural Health Care Program. HIPAA will be discussed in more detail in the following chapter relating to patient privacy.

Regulation of telemedicine in the European Union

Significant differences exist in national regulations and social security schemes across the EU, which impact the provision of telehealth services. As a result, solutions currently deployed tend to be available in single states and greater work is required to define EU-wide standards for interoperability and facilitate cross-border use. Prior to 2020, a wide gulf in telehealth utilization existed between the EU and United States. The discussion of telehealth regulations is so disparate and yet simultaneously poorly defined at a state level that it is simpler to use the US experience as a framework for discussion. While this and subsequent chapters will offer more focus on the US, EU and international perspectives will also be addressed.

The adoption of information technologies in Europe is the main accelerator of telemedicine. Prior to 2020, the telemedicine market potential has proven strong and is expected to grow at a CAGR of 14%, further driven by the adoption of wearable devices and mobile applications. Current telemedicine standards and guidelines focus primarily on technical requirements. In addition to international organizations providing guidelines, nations and EU member states also establish their own national rules. In some instances it is apparent that these rules have been created precisely for telemedicine solutions relating to a particular medical specialty. While there has been some consideration of the relevant domains of data protection, organization, human resources, ethics, and electronic health records—these are neither comprehensive nor appear to reflect joined-up thinking on the matter. Furthermore, the compatibility of standards, as an enabler for interoperability, deserves more attention, particularly if a strategic goal was to prepare for the large-scale implementation of telemedicine services.

There are concerns that current legal loopholes, including those surrounding liability and data security, will also contribute to stifle greater telehealth adoption. The EU could help address these issues in a number of ways—including through legislating for processes including a simple and workable patient consent procedure for data processing to facilitate effective collection, storage, processing, and sharing of essential health information. Presently, such activity may contravene other privacy laws in the EU which, when written, did not fully consider the needs of patients and the need for telehealth provision. The importance and significance of data protection and security should not be compromised but clearly there are different needs to be considered: where some corporations may wish to target market segments, and with sufficient granularity as to allow the identification of an individual's consumer behavior, healthcare and public health bodies may offer greater benefits to all of society through privileged access to such data. Such legislation could be introduced in a way which would not jeopardize a patient's privacy or confidentiality, but sufficient regulatory oversight and governance procedures are required. This would also require harmonization of legal frameworks and agreement on terminology and definitions. In many ways, the EU is in an advantageous position in this regard as most member states have not legislated for telehealth, and so it would be optimal for standards and definitions to be agreed upon on an EU-wide basis before codified into law at a national level.

Federal US legislation relevant to the practice of telehealth in the United States

Medicare Telehealth Services Flexibility Act (MTSFA)

The MTSFA is a bill that was introduced in the United States House of Representatives in March 2020 during the COVID-19 pandemic. The bill aimed to expand Medicare coverage for telehealth services. The MTSFA allows Medicare beneficiaries to receive telehealth services from any provider, regardless of location, as long as the provider is licensed in the state in which the patient resides. Many of the flexibilities proposed by this bill were permitted in response to there being a declared public health emergency. As a result, these flexibilities would expire once the public health emergency is over.

CARES Act

The Coronavirus Preparedness and Response Supplemental Appropriations Act became law on March 6, 2020. It not only provided healthcare agencies with additional funding to address the COVID-19 outbreak, but also eased existing telehealth restrictions in order to enhance patient access to care services. By March 17, 2020, the Centers for Medicare and Medicaid Services announced that they would expand the waiver for telehealth in several areas, including the care of new patients for issues unrelated to the public health emergency. However, this legislation did not open up telehealth billing to new practitioners. On March 27, 2020, the "Coronavirus Aid, Relief, and Economic Security Act" (CARES Act) was passed. Along with provisions centered on shoring up the economy and providing additional support for medical response, CARES includes additional funding and flexibility for telehealth provision—including giving authority to the Secretary of the Department of HHS to waive any Social Security Act provision that impedes patient care delivered by telehealth. Some of the regulations which the Secretary of the HHS has waived give insight into many of the existing barriers to the adoption of telehealth and also provide a to-do list for legislators and advocates of telehealth. These include:

- Originating site: The Secretary has waived the requirement that a beneficiary must travel to an actual site of care to receive telehealth services and has instead allowed beneficiaries to receive services wherever they are. The Secretary has also waived the geographical site restrictions on Medicare telehealth services to allow all areas and locations within the country delivery of these services, including patients' homes.
- Device type: As mentioned briefly above, it is permitted for telehealth services to be offered through personal phones and tablets, using third party applications, as long as the person receiving the service has audio and visual access to the clinician. While this is a flagrant violation of HIPAA rules, those offenders will not be fined during the public health emergency.
- Patient and service eligibility: Telehealth services have been expanded to include a wider range of services, and new patients can now use telehealth. Previously, telehealth was only available to patients who had received telehealth services from the provider within the past three years. The changes require informed consent and beneficiary initiation of the encounter but significantly increase the number of patients who can take advantage of telehealth services.
- High-deductible healthcare plans (where patients have to pay thousands of dollars before their insurance provides coverage): Access barriers and the requirement to satisfy the deductible before patients could access telehealth and risk their eligibility for health savings accounts were removed by the Secretary of HHS for the duration of the public health emergency.

As mentioned already, many of these issues still require the passing of post-pandemic legislation.

Federal communication commission's rural health care program

The FCC's Rural Health Care Program includes the Telecommunications Program and the Healthcare Connect Fund (HCF) Program. In 1996, Congress instructed the FCC to use the Universal Service Fund (USF) to provide support for both telecommunications and advanced telecommunications and information services for eligible healthcare professionals (HCPs). This federal program provides funding to help healthcare providers in rural areas get access to high-speed internet. The program provides discounts to eligible healthcare providers on their monthly broadband bills. HCPs use these services to provide telemedicine, send medical records, and perform other telemedicine activities—improving patient care—and are intended to help reduce healthcare costs.

Established in 1997, the Telecommunications Program ensures that eligible rural HCPs pay no more than their urban counterparts for telecommunication services used for healthcare purposes. The telecommunications program pays the difference between urban and rural rates for telecommunication services for eligible rural health professionals. The HCF program, launched in 2012, supports broadband connectivity and broadband networks for eligible HCPs with a 65% discount on the cost of advanced telecommunications and information services, and equipment for healthcare purposes. Support for the Rural Health Care Program was capped at $571 million per funding year subject to annual review for inflationary increases (Consumer and Government Affairs Bureau of FCC, 2019).

While this is certainly a step in the right direction, the program really only helps providers get access, and not patients, who also need to have access and are almost certainly going to be located in more rural locations than providers who often offer services from a health center. Initiatives to address disparities in access and ensuring those most in need can get affordable access to telecommunication services and equipment would not necessarily require additional public money, but in much the same way that large urban areas receive the bulk of physical infrastructure funding, which is financed by government spending, the bulk of federal telecommunication spending could be dedicated to providing rural access, where it is unprofitable for private industry to install infrastructure, and leave the infrastructure costs required in urban areas to private providers who will ultimately reap most of their profits from those markets.

Federal communications commission rules governing telehealth provision in the United States

There are four main requirements for telehealth under the FCC:

1. That patients have access to the same quality of care via telehealth as they would in person;
2. That telehealth services are provided by qualified providers;
3. That telehealth services are HIPAA compliant; and
4. That patients have the right to choose whether or not to receive care via telehealth.

While each of these sounds sensible, it is already the case that metrics such as "quality" are sufficiently nebulous as to facilitate for-profit, telehealth only organizations to seemingly satisfy these criteria, without ever having offered patients the option of in-person care, or having objectively audited the quality of care provided versus an accepted benchmark.

Requirements for telehealth

Outside of the pandemic-era waivers requested by the AMA and FSMB to reduce telehealth requirements, there are several key focus areas of state telehealth laws.

Licensing

Licensing requirements for HCPs can vary between jurisdictions. Broadly speaking, telehealth services in the United States are regulated by state laws and professional licensure boards. Each state has its own regulations governing the provision of telehealth services, and these regulations can vary significantly from state to state. It is not a case of the physician being licensed in the state in which they practice telehealth, but rather, in many cases, the provider must currently adhere to licensing requirements in the state in which the patient is located during the encounter. In general, however, telehealth providers must be licensed in the state in which they are providing services. Some states have enacted laws that specifically address the provision of telehealth services. These laws may exempt telehealth providers from certain licensure requirements, or they may establish specific licensure requirements for telehealth providers. Other states have not enacted specific legislation governing telehealth, but licensure requirements for telehealth providers may be included in general laws governing the practice of medicine or the delivery of healthcare services.

In addition to state licensure requirements, telehealth providers must also comply with federal laws and regulations, including the HIPAA (which is discussed in more detail in the following chapter of this book) and the FCC rules governing the use of telecommunications equipment and services.

Medical malpractice insurance

This depends on the insurer, but expect that it's less likely and more difficult when care across states is being provided. This is not just suggesting that a physician is caring for patients from a different country, but also considers a patient that is no longer in the country where the medical relationship was established—a patient could be anywhere and seek a medical consult from you online. In such an instance, consider which countries' laws matter and with which regulatory bodies the practitioner should be registered.

Clinician—patient relationship

The definition of the clinician—patient relationship varies between jurisdictions and now contexts: in person versus telehealth. The physician—patient relationship is defined by some as a professional relationship between a licensed physician and a patient within which the physician provides medical care and services to the patient. Others extend this definition, describing it as a contract between a physician and a patient in which the physician agrees to provide medical care and advice to the patient in exchange for the patient's agreement to follow the physician's instructions.

In the context of telehealth though, some jurisdictions require that a relationship be established first by an in-person visit before telehealth sessions can be conducted, while others believe that an effective clinician–patient relationship can be established by leveraging telehealth technology. In other words, in some jurisdictions, patients may never meet their physician in person, yet receive care from them.

Online prescribing

There are strict compliance requirements in place in some jurisdictions for prescribing medications online, with some requiring an in-person visit before certain types of medications can be prescribed. There is a chapter focused on e-prescribing later in this book.

It is also important to note that in the EU, Directive 2011/24/EU ensures the recognition of prescriptions issued in another member state, how to identify the medicine prescribed (where drug designation may vary between states) and how to identify the prescriber. It should be noted that this directive only applies to telemedicine operating beyond national boundaries, where patient and physician are both resident within the EU. When telemedicine operates within national boundaries, this Directive does not apply, since the regulation of healthcare delivery within a state rests with that state.

Informed consent

Some jurisdictions require written informed consent before conducting telehealth services. While this legal requirement is not universal, there are moral and ethical considerations that must be taken into account. Informed consent is the process through which a patient is made aware of the risks, benefits, and alternatives to a proposed treatment and provides their permission to proceed. Informed consent is a cornerstone of ethical healthcare and is necessary to protect the rights of patients. When providing care via telehealth, it is advisable to obtain informed consent from patients prior to providing care. This can be done through the use of a consent form that is signed by the patient or through an electronic process that documents the patient's consent. There are several reasons why informed consent is even more important when providing care via telehealth. First, patients may be more likely to experience anxiety and feelings of vulnerability when receiving care via telehealth. This is due to the fact that they are not physically present with the provider, and may feel additional anxiety over the use of technology or devices which they do not feel comfortable with or in control of, which can compound a situation where a patient may find it difficult to understand what is happening.

Additionally, and while I am not an advocate for the practice of defensive medicine, informed consent helps to protect providers from liability in the event that something goes wrong during the course of treatment. Informed consent is critical when providing telehealth services. Without it, patients may not be fully aware of the risks and benefits of the treatment and may not be able to make an informed decision about whether or not to proceed with it. Informed consent forms should therefore be clear and concise and should explain the risks and benefits of the treatment in plain language. Patients should be given ample time to read and understand the form before being asked to sign it and should be provided with a copy of the document for their own records.

Reimbursement and telehealth billing and payments

Private payers and Medicaid reimbursement vary significantly between states. Where full reimbursement is available for some, others take a tiered reimbursement approach and have outlined which services are covered and which are not. There are exceptions to all of these general guidelines. For example, the Department of Veteran Affairs (VA) issued a rule in 2018 which allows VA healthcare providers to provide care in any state, regardless of the provider's and patient's location.

Challenges existed long before the public health emergency, and some are beyond the reach of the Secretary of HHS and existing legislation. Some of the barriers to telehealth payments related to federal programs and private insurers, while others exist because of payment processors, the digital payment and electronic fund transfer systems and agreements that private industry has imposed on healthcare providers.

CMS payment issues

Since March 30, 2020, under temporary provisions, the CMS, using section 1135 of the Social Security Act, issued a blanket waiver allowing flexible billing provisions for telehealth, which again are for the duration of the public health emergency period. Medicare and Medicaid are the federally administered health coverage plans for older, disabled, and low-income individuals in the United States, which accounts for over 100 million people or almost one in three Americans. These temporary waivers are therefore a huge opportunity for telehealth providers to demonstrate the utility of this technology and telehealth services, so that when the temporary waivers expire, there is an easy win for legislators looking to help reduce the cost of health services in the United States (which now stands at over $4.1 trillion) and help improve health outcomes, a category in which the United States of America ranks last among high-income nations (Kuehn, 2021).

Despite the huge opportunity, an issue that has long existed, and that will again offer a barrier to telehealth services if formal legislation does not address them, is that audio-only telehealth services did not satisfy the definition of using interactive telecommunications systems to furnish two-way, real-time audio and video health services, as video services were not offered. This may become less of an issue as patients get greater access to, and become more familiar with, video consult services and operating smart devices and allowing requisite hardware permissions so as to complete a video and audio call.

Requirements for hospitals and critical access hospitals related to telemedicine were waived by CMS along with many other seemingly small pieces of information, which in sum would make meaningful practice near impossible. For example, CMS requires details of home health aides, skilled nursing facilities, inpatient rehabilitation facilities, and long-term care hospitals available to the patient to be disclosed prior to discharge from care from an health facility as well as needing physicians to be physically present to provide medical direction, consultation, or supervision of services for patients. If an institution had not built out such information and infrastructure to facilitate these processes for digital health provision, then they would be unable to provide the service.

Telemedicine coverage and payments for such services vary widely. While public and private tax payers continue to develop formal payment mechanisms for telemedicine services, there are still inconsistencies and these act as barriers to the further spread of telemedicine. Outside of emergency time waivers, Medicare provides payment to physicians and other health professionals for a very limited list of Part B services (Part B incorporates two services: medically necessary services like services and supplies needed to diagnose and treat a medical condition and preventative services including early diagnosis and vaccination efforts, and so incorporates things from durable medical equipment through to outpatient health visits and outpatient prescription drugs). Prior to the temporary emergency procedures to allow nationwide access to telehealth, only payment for some telehealth services was available in 47 of the 50 US states; only 16 states had programs in place to pay for remote patient monitoring. Less than half of US states (23) had laws mandating that private insurers cover what the states deem as telemedicine services with differing definitions (American Medical Association, 2015).

Payment processing providers

Payment processing providers do not universally provide their services to healthcare clinics. To be clear, many providers of gateway services required to process a payment from a credit or debit card, like you would in a restaurant or supermarket, and who charge a base fee and percentage of the transaction for their services, are not willing to accept physicians or healthcare practices as customers. This will be discussed elsewhere in this book, but briefly, the current behemoths of online and digital payment systems (Stripe, PayPal) specifically exclude health providers as customers, and those that do accept licensed healthcare providers are often compelled by their own providers to charge higher fees sometimes as a result of contract-level agreements and also as a risk premium and to offset the high rate of payment chargebacks, which they state the sector has traditionally received.

Infrastructure

In the same way that patient care in a brick-and-mortar practice requires HCPs sharing information and interacting with each other using a common language, vocabulary and set of care standards, telehealth requires the same. Multiple infrastructure components are required to successfully implement telehealth services, including systems that operate using standards of interoperability, compliance, and individuals who have received adequate training to operate them. Often this may require the development and institution of practice protocols. While exact technical infrastructure requirements depend on the type of telemedicine services that one plans to offer, nearly all telemedicine programs require the following:

Internet access

High-speed reliable broadband internet access will minimize provider-side internet glitches and ensure stable and reliable transmission of quality video and audio, helping to facilitate productive consultations. Nobody wants to have their call dropped or have poor audio quality during a consultation. The provider can do little to control connectivity issues of the patient, but bandwidth limitations are becoming less and less of an issue with more widespread availability of high-quality internet service providers. Where wires and cell towers do not reach, there is greater availability of satellite internet providers such as Viasat and Starlink, which are satellite internet providers focused on private consumers, and not just larger corporations, and as such, aim to provide the service at a price point accessible to many, and not just the few.

While internet service providers are keen to advertise maximum and theoretical speeds that their service could provide, they often do not clearly state the realistic speeds obtained, nor the contention ratio. A contention ratio is the number of people sharing a connection at any given time. The higher the contention ratio, the slower the connection will be. Most residential broadband providers have a contention ratio of 50:1, which means that 50 people are sharing the same connection at the same time. This can significantly impact not just the average bandwidth but also the quality of an uploaded and downloaded high-quality, audio and video stream. Generally speaking, business connections provide lower contention ratios, but ultimately, the experience is also reliant on the connection utilized by the patient.

Technical support

The provision of healthcare relies upon the integrity of the tools utilized in its provision. If hardware or software issues arise, it can disable the practice from being able to confidently provide telehealth services. Rapid and robust technical support is required to remediate any issues that may arise and not compromise patient care. This is particularly important during any phase where new staff members may join the practice team and not just during the initial setup and rollout of a telehealth service.

Practices should anticipate not just their own technical support needs, but also those of their patients. Much in the same way as social history is important for caring for all patients, in the era of telehealth, technological factors are too, and should be considered before scheduling a telehealth consult for a patient. These will be discussed in more detail in the patient considerations chapter.

Digital imaging/cameras and microphones

These devices allow providers and patients to see and communicate with each other. While many cameras come with inbuilt microphones, depending on the context of one's medical practice, dedicated high-quality audio equipment helps reduce patient frustrations and reduce background noise.

Supplemental telehealth technology

While in-person visits to a healthcare provider's office often include hands-on tasks such as measuring the pulse or blood pressure of a patient, telehealth visits can achieve the same through the use of reliable remote measurements from blood pressure cuffs, two lead electrocardiograms, or digital stethoscopes.

Training

Urologists, in particular, are familiar with the learning curves associated with the adoption of new technologies, devices, and surgical systems. Likewise, the efficiencies promised by telehealth will only be fully realized when providers and patients can use them effectively. Training in telehealth (for both patients and healthcare providers) and the use of patient-friendly systems are essential to achieve this.

Patient requirements

While it may sound obvious, ensuring both the patient and the consultation are suitable for telehealth is essential. People often have preconceptions about technology—thinking it can do things it can't, or that it's doing things it isn't. Ensuring your patient is able and willing to engage with connected devices and be prepared for digital visits is key for successful telehealth care delivery. Preparing patients for telehealth is discussed further later in the book.

Bibliography

American Medical Association. (2015). *Coverage and payment for telemedicine* [Press release]. Retrieved from https://www.ama-assn.org/sites/ama-assn.org/files/corp/media-browser/premium/arc/coverage-of-and-payment-for-telemedicine-issue-brief_0.pdf.

Consumer and Government Affairs Bureau of FCC. (2019). *The FCC's universal service rural health care program.* Retrieved from http://www.fcc.gov/consumer-governmental-affairs-bureau.

Kuehn, B. M. (2021). US health system ranks last among high-income countries. *The Journal of the American Medical Association, 326*(11), 999. https://doi.org/10.1001/jama.2021.15468

https://www.cms.gov/files/document/covid-19-emergency-declaration-waivers.pdf.

Patient privacy laws

Introduction

A core principle upon which medicine is practiced is that of trust, specifically between patient and physician. And key to that trust is not betraying a patient's fundamental human rights—including the right to privacy. It is worth acknowledging that contemporary surveys of patients suggest they are not worried about the confidentiality of their private information being exchanged through telemedicine (Adams et al., 2021). A similar impression is shared by physicians, but empirical evidence suggests that all involved parties are overconfident in the security of such systems and devices.

Many would consider this to be a very clear-cut topic, where there exist Federal laws in the United States, European Union (EU)-wide laws, and other states with defined privacy laws, governing data handling and or patient privacy. However, this is not the case. For healthcare providers handling any patient details, protected health information (PHI), or otherwise, it is worth knowing that some such laws currently do not apply to every patient seeking care, and that some practices, may knowingly, or unknowingly be the source of data used for the exploitation of those same patients. Many, while informed, are not conscious that credit card and other payment providers have granular data on who you are, what doctors you pay with your credit card or other digital payment solution, and how much you spend at the pharmacy counter versus how much you spend on confectionary, cosmetics, or other product categories at the pharmacy. Considering this data repository is longitudinal and long term for many, inference of what exact medical condition, its status, and other details of health conditions can be made with high fidelity. These data points are legally available for purchase from these payment providers, by anyone willing to pay. And many do purchase this information.

A general approach where all patient information should be treated as PHI, and in the same way, for telemedicine consults as it would be for in person visits, is reasonable. However, what might not be so obvious is that by practicing telehealth, there likely are other measures and protocols that should be followed to protect patient information. The famed Health Insurance Portability and Accountability Act

Telehealth in Urology. https://doi.org/10.1016/B978-0-323-87480-9.00008-7

(HIPAA) which passed in congress in 1996 is not all encompassing. It is famed as giving patients' control over their information such as the right to examine and obtain records, and it is the US national standard to protect medical records and other personal health information. It applies to health plans, healthcare clearinghouses, and healthcare providers but only those who receive reimbursement from federal sources. To be explicit, private practices do not have any legal requirement to abide by HIPAA and are not prevented from sharing, selling, or otherwise disclosing patient health information by this law.

HIPAA acts as the floor on health information. There are also state health information and privacy laws. Some states have more stringent laws in place in regards to health information. States cannot have laws that are of lesser strength or run counter to HIPAA. If they do, the federal law will prevail. However, states can have much stricter and more robust laws than HIPAA. For example, the State of California has the California Confidentiality of Medical Information Act (CMIA). On the surface, CMIA is a state law that requires healthcare providers to maintain the confidentiality of their patients' medical information. The CMIA also prohibits healthcare providers from disclosing medical information without the patient's written consent. It is worth noting that it does not prohibit the third parties such as payment providers from disclosing information. On the other hand, CMIA's definitions are much broader than HIPAA—including for "provider of healthcare" and "all recipients of healthcare."

The issue of the location of the provider and the location of the patient is critical again. The applicability of these laws, both federal and regional, does not change because you are using telehealth. Location does not shield from HIPAA or other privacy laws which would normally apply. While the general guideline is to treat a telehealth consult no different than an in person visit, additional safeguards also need to be taken. A simple example is that in the provision of telehealth, providers may use services from vendors that they would not ordinarily use as part of their practice where they see patients who physically present. Examples include using a short message service/text messaging service, or a video consult service—where one would need to meet legal requirements such as specific contracts or a business associate agreement with them in order to be compliant with HIPAA or other relevant legislation.

Potential privacy risks

Lack of control or lack of limits on the collection, use, and disclosure of sensitive personal information is a potential privacy risk of telehealth, and indeed the connected home in general. Sensors or devices that are located in a patient's home, whether or not they interface with the patient's body may also have the capacity to collect sensitive information about household activities, which offer a potential opportunity to improve healthcare monitoring, but also risk invading personal privacy.

Devices explicitly made for health purposes may also transmit information, which can disclose or allow other personal and private information to be deduced. Consider sensors used to detect falls; these can transmit information which would provide religious practices or intimate interactions or indeed even indicate when nobody is at home. Whatever about the use of the information by the health provider, the presence of the device maybe because of the provider aiming to provide telehealth. Much like a provider will discuss the risks and benefits of any other potential investigation, intervention, or treatment with a patient, such devices also carry their own risks and benefits.

The routine transmission from such devices used in the investigation, intervention, or treatment of a medical condition may also be collected and stored by the device, or app, or its manufacturer, or shared with third parties. Consider, for example, that many mobile applications, (e.g., the Facebook app) currently collect information on the presence of what other apps are installed on your device, and when they run. Such collection, use and disclosure of information may be beyond what patients reasonably expect given anticipated uses of the technology. This happened in the case of a popular fitness device inadvertently exposing user's self-reported sexual activity.

This brings to the fore an ethical responsibility of physicians: nonmaleficence. Patients may give consent to have a device implanted, or to wear sensors and be tracked, or to use a health app and share their data. However, consent should not abrogate the universal human right to privacy. All of us frequently do not read or fully understand privacy policies. How many people have actually read the privacy policies of the company's services we use online every day? Patients place their trust in physicians to care for them and to bring no harm to them. Some use consent as a tool to shift the burden of privacy protection to the patient, who may not be able to make meaningful privacy choices.

Privacy controls in the USA

Privacy is typically protected by laws or operating policies that implement Fair Information Practice Principles (FIPPs). FIPPs are widely accepted practices, including the ability to access one's own health information and request corrections; limitations on information collection, use, and disclosure; and reasonable opportunities to make choices about one's own health information. Providing people with choices for information sharing is only one of the FIPPs, bolstered by others that require data holders to establish and abide by contextually appropriate limits on data access, use, and disclosure.

HIPAA

The HIPAA of 1996 is one of several sectoral federal laws designed to implement these principles. Current laws, however, do not adequately cover the telehealth environment. Thus, there is no guaranteed right (and often little capability) for individuals to request copies of information collected by apps or home monitoring devices. Information use and disclosure are largely determined by technology companies, with few (if any) legal limits or meaningful opportunities for individuals to control information flow.

HIPAA privacy and security regulations provide protections for identifiable health information, but only when it is collected and shared by "covered entities"— healthcare providers who bill electronically using HIPAA standards, health plans, and healthcare clearinghouses. When it applies, HIPAA's Privacy Rule establishes limits on the use and disclosure of identifiable health information, and its Security Rule establishes technical, physical, and administrative safeguards to be adopted to protect electronic identifiable health information. For example, encryption of data at rest and in transit is an "addressable implementation specification" under the Security Rule, meaning that HIPAA-covered entities are expected to implement it unless it is not "reasonable and appropriate" to do so. In addition, the regulation states, providers are required to adopt identity management protocols and access controls.

HITECH Act 2009

The Health Information Technology for Economic and Clinical Health (HITECH) Act of 2009 saw the US Congress extend HIPAA to "business associates," entities that "create, receive, maintain, or transmit" identifiable health information to perform a function or service "on behalf of" a covered entity. Whether a vendor of a patient-facing telehealth technology is a HIPAA business associate depends on whose interests are being served by the technology. Relevant questions include the following: Who provides the technology to the patient (for example, is it a direct-to-patient transaction, or is the technology provided by the doctor)? Who benefits from the technology being offered? Who is responsible for the day-to-day operation of the technology (an indication of who is ultimately responsible)? And who controls the information generated by the technology? Mere connectivity between a device and a healthcare provider does not render the device manufacturer a business associate of that provider.

Federal trade commission regulations

HIPAA has limited applicability to patient-facing telehealth systems. The HITECH Act established breach notification requirements for personal health records. The requirements of this are overseen by the Federal Trade Commission (FTC). This is probably one of the least well-appreciated and possibly one of the greatest privacy protections offered to patients and users of digital tools. The HITECH Act defines a "personal health record" as an electronic record of identifiable information "drawn from multiple sources and … manage, shared, and controlled" by the patient. While many telehealth tools will not meet this definition, as they don't draw information from multiple sources and most are not typically controlled by the patient, one can see how application data from social media applications can be defined as "personal health records," where the information is identifiable, drawn from multiple sources, and it is managed, shared, and controlled (at least in part) by the patient.

The FTC Act allows the FTC to seek redress for unfair or deceptive acts or practices. The FTC has used this authority frequently to penalize companies for failing to abide by commitments regarding data use made in privacy policies and less frequently to stop unfair practices involving data use and collection. Users of digital apps must rely on the company policy regarding use of data, which are almost always offered to users unilaterally. In other words: if you don't accept the terms, you don't use the product or service. Unfortunately, in the case of medical devices, patients often do not have a choice.

Oversight by the FDA

If a telehealth technology qualifies as a medical device, the Food and Drug Administration (FDA) may also regulate it. The FDA does not directly address privacy issues but focuses on security to the extent that it affects medical device safety. (The FDA regulation of mobile medical apps is discussed in greater detail elsewhere in this publication.) In June 2013, the FDA issued draft guidance on the "management of cybersecurity in medical devices," which urges manufacturers to develop security controls to maintain information "confidentiality, integrity, and availability." In August 2013, the FDA finalized guidance regarding radio frequency wireless technology in medical devices. And in September 2013, the FDA issued broad guidance on the regulation of mobile medical apps, clarifying that some types of mobile medical apps will be considered medical devices and regulated by the FDA as such.

Through these guidance documents, the FDA is establishing a federal baseline for security in telehealth, but the FDA's authority has limits. The FDA oversees only technologies it considers to be medical devices and focuses only on security protections designed to ensure safety. It does not focus on privacy safeguards that enforce rules or policies regarding collection, use, and disclosure of potentially sensitive health information.

There will ultimately be further privacy laws implemented, so watch this space

A comprehensive federal policy framework protecting the privacy and security of information collected by telehealth technologies is needed to safeguard patients and bolster public trust. Such protections should be consistent with the basic tenets of HIPAA to ensure a rational and predictable policy environment, but they also should respond to threats to privacy and security that are more characteristic of patient- and consumer-facing technologies. Specifically, policy should address issues such as deficiencies in security safeguards, reliance by app companies on advertising within the apps, and consumers' lack of access to their information. It should account for current and potential future sources of data leaks, which are de facto sources of identifiable health information, and help close loopholes (or the vast chasms) in existing legislation, which allow for patient information to be shared. Such policies should be tailored to address the unique telehealth risks we have identified here. The policies should cover data collection, use, and disclosure, for both the intended purpose of the technology and any secondary data uses, such as for analytics. They should also be flexible enough to support innovation.

There are a number of challenges to crafting such a policy framework. Privacy and security concerns sometimes can conflict with practicality for patients and industry. Privacy and security controls that do not anticipate the needs and preferences of the intended users are less likely to be deployed. For example, Apple (now the world's largest company by market capitalization) discovered that only half of iPhone users lock their devices with a passcode. Apple, in essence acknowledging the potential risk to an individual by not locking their phone, made a costly decision to integrate a fingerprint reader into newer models of the iPhone to make it easier to lock the device, and subsequently integrating facial recognition to unlock devices; perhaps a defensive move by Apple, whereby they took all practical steps possible to make it easier for users to secure their information and opting out of security that was easy to use and readily available.

An uneasy balance between operational practicality, privacy and security is not unique to healthcare. It exists in banking and telecommunications also, and whatever about millennia old banking, it is damning that telecommunications have done more to address this than healthcare. Consider the Cable TV Privacy Act of 1984 and the Telecommunications Act of 1996, which prevent the disclosure of personal information without consent and also provide protections akin to FIPPs. These act to balance the business and operational needs of cable and telecommunications providers by allowing the sharing of personal information if the customer fails to opt out of such sharing and are really nothing more than a regulatory loophole, which has social implications and allows for-profit enterprises to exploit individuals information for further profit (Rogers Jr, 1980). In banking, the Fair Credit Reporting Act of 1970 and the Gramm–Leach–Bliley Act of 1999 heavily regulate what credit reporting agencies and financial services companies can do with personal information, providing for conspicuous and regular notice of privacy practices and rights of correction and transparency for consumers. However, these laws also favor an opt-out approach for sharing personal information—allowing data to flow by default to other companies unless the customer specifically opts out, opening the door to selling individual-level user information (Code, 1999; Hall & McGraw, 2014).

No federal agency currently has the authority to establish privacy and security requirements for the telehealth industry. However, the US Congress could pass legislation that would vest this authority with a single federal agency. The Department of Health and Human Services (HHS) is a likely candidate for this role, as it already has experience implementing the HIPAA privacy rules and overseeing US health programs. However, HHS does not have any experience with the privacy and security risks posed by consumer-facing commercial technologies. Another possible agency for this role is the FDA, which is responsible for ensuring the safety of telehealth devices. However, the FDA does not have any experience with privacy issues. On the other hand, the FTC—part of the US Department of Commerce—has technical expertise and long experience in evaluating the privacy risks of consumer-facing technologies. Some would argue it is the agency within the federal government most equipped to regulate information privacy, including within networked tele-health systems.

With respect to telehealth, US Congress could give the FTC authority and build on the Department of Commerce's 2010 outline for "voluntary enforceable codes of conduct" with respect to consumer privacy (Department of Commerce, 2010). The development of voluntary codes of conduct by telehealth manufacturers and other stakeholders, including those that represent the interests of individual innovators and also healthcare professionals, could be facilitated by the FTC or whichever agency ultimately is granted oversight. These codes of conduct should include foundational privacy and security protections at a minimum. As telehealth continues to rapidly evolve, continuous and equitable involvement of stakeholders in further developing these codes of conduct is critical. The FTC of course already has existing authority to regulate deceptive and unfair practices, and so is well placed to enforce such protections and use carrot and stick strategies. For example, through financial penalties and other means, compel manufacturers to adopt them and on the other hand, induce industry to develop and adopt these codes of conduct by granting a safe harbor from enforcement action for those activities governed by the codes. To provide meaningful protection, Safe Harbor should only be granted to codes that the FTC deems adequate to protect consumers (Hall & McGraw, 2014).

While the absence of a perfect agency will surely stifle agreement and implementation, it shouldn't. It is in patients' best interests that such oversight is in place regardless of whomever is bestowed this responsibility, and it is imperative that they be agile, innovative, and sufficiently informed to respond to privacy and technology concerns, first protecting patients but doing so without stifling innovation or implementation in this space. Ultimately though, policy makers need to take action to place meaningful patient protections in place, as once this information is in the hands of public corporations or private entities, clawing it back will be near impossible.

European regulations and laws

Patient privacy in the EU is governed by a number of laws and regulations, which establish strict rules on how personal data must be collected, used, and protected. Individuals in the EU have a legal right to know what personal data are being collected about them, the right to have that data erased or corrected, and the right to object to its use, including a "right to be forgotten." Many of these laws and regulations are general privacy laws and apply to healthcare as they do to all sectors, and so in many respects are less prone to loopholes and strategies to sidestep regulations than if they were only applicable to the provision of health, which is in anyway reimbursed by the government.

GDPR—general data protection regulation

The EU through legislation and other efforts aims to address current and impending challenges in the practice and adoption of telehealth, as there are numerous legal, regulatory, and interoperability challenges. A common eHealth framework has been developed (eHealth EU Interoperability Framework). The EU is also aiming to ensure incidents of data misuse by commercial entities including those based outside of the EU are prevented and that a balance be struck between protecting citizens and facilitating medical innovation.

GDPR was introduced in 2016 and became applicable across all member states of the EU on May 25, 2018. GDPR is widely considered to have a broader scope of effect than HIPAA does in the United States of America. The objectives of GDPR are:

1. to facilitate free movement of personal data, including cross-border exchange and
2. to protect the fundamental rights and freedoms of natural persons with regard to privacy and protection of personal data (Article 1 of GDPR).

There is a fundamental challenge though to the protection of personal privacy in eHealth when digital devices are used: it is often possible to reidentify a person even from "anonymized data" through the combination of metadata, which form a unique digital signature of that user.

Data protection directive—passed October 24, 1995

The EU Data Protection Directive is a set of regulations that member states of the EU must implement in order to protect the privacy of digital data. The directive was passed in 1995 and updated in 2018. It requires member states to provide subjects with the right to access their personal data, the right to rectify inaccurate data, and the right to data portability. It also establishes rules for data processors, such as requiring them to implement security measures to protect data and to only process data for specified purposes. Finally, the directive creates a mechanism for subjects to file complaints with national data protection authorities. The EU Data Protection Directive sets out strict rules about how personal data must be collected, used, and protected.

Personal data must be:

- Legitimate and necessary for the purposes for which it is being used.
- Accurately and carefully collected.
- Used only for the purposes for which it was collected and not used for any other purpose.
- Erased or destroyed if it is no longer needed and is not being used for any other purpose.
- Protected against unauthorized or accidental access, destruction, alteration, or unauthorized use.

However, this directive allows for the processing of health data without explicit consent. For example, article 8(3) of the Data Protection Directive permits processing by a health professional subject to confidentiality rules for the purposes of preventive medicine, medical diagnosis, the provision of care or treatment, or the management of healthcare services. The other main weaknesses of the EU Data Protection Directive are that it does not provide for a private right of action, it does not apply to non-EU data controllers, and it does not have a mechanism for enforcing data protection rights.

EU e-privacy directive

The EU e-privacy directive was introduced on May 25, 2018. It is a regulation that requires websites to obtain consent from users before collecting or using their personal data. The directive applies to all electronic communications, including email, instant messaging, telephone calls, and internet use. It requires that electronic communications service providers take measures to protect the confidentiality of communications and gives users the right to access their communications data. The regulation also requires websites to provide users with clear and concise information about their data collection and use practices.

The directive covers a wide range of topics, including the use of cookies, spam, and unsolicited communications. The directive is a strong piece of legislation that provides robust protections for the privacy of electronic communications. It is also flexible, allowing member states to tailor the implementation of the directive to their own national laws and regulations.

For all of its positives, there are also a number of limitations of the directive:

- It is not well-defined, and there is significant confusion over what it actually covers.
- It is not enforced consistently, and there are significant loopholes that allow companies to avoid compliance.
- It does not cover all types of data, including some types that are particularly sensitive (e.g., financial data).
- It does not provide for adequate penalties for companies that violate the directive.
- It does not allow individuals to effectively opt out of having their data collected and used.

The directive has also been criticized for its vague and imprecise language and for its potential to conflict with other EU directives, such as the e-commerce directive.

Conclusions

Trust is at the center of the patient—doctor relationship. Lapses in patient privacy erode this trust and irreversibly damage this relationship. To establish greater trust in telehealth and facilitate more meaningful adoption of the promises of telemedicine, health information security which ensures privacy must be prioritized. Stakeholders should seek to implement a comprehensive framework, which accommodates the detail and flexibility needed for the evolving complexities of providing telehealth and e-health services. There is as much patient education as physician education required to secure and ensure privacy of health data. While statutory direction already exists, it is all too quickly made redundant by the successes of e-health innovators and visionaries. It is difficult to differentiate between well-intentioned innovators and predatory profiteers, but patient privacy is too precious to risk, even for the potential rewards of a fully realized e-health system.

Bibliography

Adams, R. B., Nelson, V. R., & Holtz, B. E. (2021). Barriers for telemedicine use among non-users at the beginning of the pandemic. *Telemedicine Reports, 2*(1), 211–216. https://doi.org/10.1089/tmr.2021.0022

Code, U. (1999). Gramm-leach-bliley act. In *Gramm-leach-bliley act/AHIMA*. American Health Information Management Association.

Department of Commerce. (2010). *Commercial data privacy and innovation in the internet economy: A dynamic policy framework*. Washington D.C. Retrieved from https://www.ntia.doc.gov https://www.ntia.doc.gov/report/2010/commercial-data-privacy-and-innovation-internet-economy-dynamic-policy-framework.

Hall, J. L., & McGraw, D. (2014). For telehealth to succeed, privacy and security risks must be identified and addressed. *Health Affairs, 33*(2), 216–221. https://doi.org/10.1377/hlthaff.2013.0997

Rogers, W. A., Jr. (1980). Repealing section 222 of the communications act. *Texas Law Review, 59*, 559.

https://telehealthtechnology.org/= national telehealth technology assessment resource center ((USA)).

https://www.cchpca.org/?s=privacy.

How do I get started providing a telehealth service?

2

Getting started in telehealth

Introduction

Incorporating telemedicine into your practice is not a one-size-fits-all solution. Preconceived notions of what telemedicine is or what it should be may prevent many from venturing further. Technological complexity and the number of technologies that are available will likely continue to follow a trend similar to Moore's law, (that the number of transistors on microchips will double approximately every two years, and that technology will become faster, smaller and more efficient as time passes). Planning for the provision of telehealth and predicting what exact technologies will next reach prime time in healthcare seems an arduous task; but there is a useful rubric or list which can be used, to help the urology practice deciding how to plan their telemedicine offerings (also see Fig. 3.1):

- Teleconsults: new patients and or established patient consultations
- Digital diagnostics
- Telemonitoring or remote care
- Wellness monitoring for preventive care
- Digital health interventions
- Teleprocedures

Each of these will be discussed in more detail in the coming chapters but briefly; teleconsultation or teleconsults are considered by some to be "hands-free" medicine. They are considered by some to be most suited for follow-up encounters rather than initial encounters; however, this need not be the case for every type of consult. While the importance of physical examination to clinical medicine can and should never be diminished, there is growing commentary that suggests it is often neglected in modern medicine, and telehealth offerings will likely add further to this trend as they have not yet solved for this. The point of saying this is that a useful starting point is to consider which patients, which physicians, and which consults are most appropriate and perhaps better served by a teleconsult. This work can begin with a simple audit of visits, or survey of patients at your clinic, to establish if patients would have been happy to have completed their visit, or their next visit by a teleconsult. This is a low effort but high-return activity and will better prepare both practice and patients for such a service. A study from the Department of Urology in a Veteran Affairs

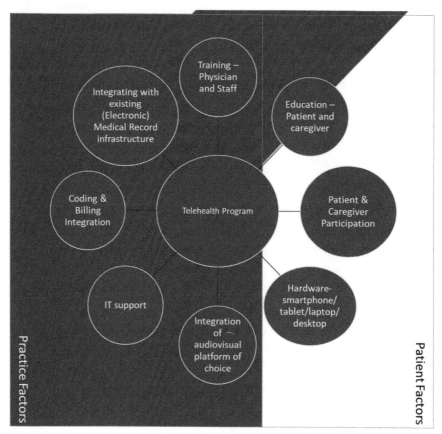

FIGURE 3.1

Graphical representation of the framework for implementation—proposed by Smith et al. (2020).

hospital in the greater Los Angeles area, which was conducted pre-COVID-19 pandemic in 2015, reported 95% of patients report their care via telehealth as "very good" to "excellent" (Chu et al., 2015).

The opportunity and the challenge

For many, telehealth has been or will be the insertion of a webcam into their consult room. It may be the insertion of a webcam into a room that wasn't intended to be a consult room, or it may be replacing the act of walking from waiting room to consult room, with a webcam—the "webcamification" of a practice. It can be so much more, and this change offers a wonderful opportunity: any practice habits that have been in need of change or improvement can now use this moment to enact this change.

Consider the practice where the workflow might see a patient approach the registration desk, meet the administrative staff member, check in, receive a clipboard of questions to complete, including demographic information, past medical history, and billing information. The patient is reseated, completes the information, before returning to the registration desk to hand off this information to the administrative staff and confirm their identity with an acceptable form of ID. The admin then reviews and transcribes the information into the electronic medical record (EMR). The patient will be called and see the practice nurse for triage, measurement of vital signs, weight, height, and collection of clinical samples, before being reseated and before finally moving to see the advanced nurse practitioner/physician assistant/physician.

Telehealth provides the opportunity to make this process more efficient: to reduce the start-stop journey of the patient on a typical clinic visit, to eliminate administrative staff transcribing information, and allow them to help verify information instead of placing them in a position where they make transcription errors.

Addressing disparities

Despite improvements in terms of access, there is a risk that telehealth can exacerbate disparities: not everyone has a reliable internet connection, or the correct tools to participate in a telehealth consult. Not everyone is comfortable or tech-literate. The solutions here are often generational, and indeed not new. Not everybody can just pop in to their local hospital; prior to telehealth, there were (and still are) vast swathes of people who did not have access to healthcare by mere virtue of proximity. Telehealth is not a prescription for distrust or mistrust of the healthcare system. It can provide a part of the solution, but it is not the panacea. Government policy and healthcare delivery will need to keep pace and evolve. Fee for service models where urologists are reimbursed only when a patient comes into the office, when the clinical team physically examines, performs a test, completes procedure, or writes a prescription will need to be reexamined. Many already find this model unfit for the purpose of improving patient's health, and the broader offering and delivery of telehealth offers the opportunity for practices, as large stakeholders in this process, to help redesign and improve the healthcare system of which they are a part.

Telehealth offers all urologists in practice with an opportunity they are not otherwise offered. Urologists can look at their practice, and design anew, how they want to provide and care for their patients; with due regard provided to those who come from a poorly served group who have had physical, language, systemic, or other barriers to their care provision.

Payments/reimbursement

While differences exist in healthcare models, much of contemporary urological telehealth prior to the COVID-19 pandemic was being offered by subscription health services offering care for preselected urological issues, such as erectile dysfunction and the medical management of lower urinary tract dysfunction and incontinence.

The service a practitioner provides need not conform to existing models requiring insurance preapproval, nor must it be a subscription model only, caring for one or a few cherry-picked urological complaints.

At present, and in part due to COVID-19 emergency health measures, reimbursement for urological care provided by telehealth is typically reimbursed by insurance companies in the same way as in-person visits. It is hoped that reimbursement in much the same way can be continued once this emergency ends. Reimbursement is discussed in more detail later in this book.

Implementation and strategy
Provider and staff training

For those confident with digital systems, and troubleshooting software and hardware issues, at least an hour of preparation and training with the various tools that will be employed for a telehealth visit is required. For those less familiar, more resources and guided education are often beneficial. Where training must end, a mock consult or training consult will give everyone the opportunity to test out the workflow, become familiar with operating systems, and help provide confidence to staff, who will in turn help troubleshoot for patients and give patients greater confidence in using new and sometimes unfamiliar technologies.

A suggestion for getting started is to have a "soft" launch, where all staff and not just providers can gain confidence and troubleshoot any issues without usual time constraints. Although telemedicine is often built as a physician platform, it is prudent to include the front desk and nursing staff within the telemedicine model to mimic a standard in-person encounter. I would suggest that for the first week or for the soft launch for inexperienced practices, all telemedicine visits are limited to 30 min for both new and return patient visits. Once familiarity and competence are demonstrated, providers can choose to adjust their clinic attendance to better accommodate patients.

Patient education

Office staff will spend time upfront to present the option of a telemedicine visit to patients and coach them through the necessary software for the first encounter. Patients will be made aware of potential advantages of the telemedicine visit such as not postponing their healthcare needs while staying safely at home, having the ability to save travel and waiting times, and avoiding the expenses associated with transportation and parking. I would suggest nursing staff should call patients approximately one week ahead of their appointment to confirm their preferred method of audiovisual communication or that they are prepared to use the platform your practice prefers to use. It's also useful that they explain the procedures ahead of time so patients are prepared.

Further, I would suggest that shortly before the scheduled telemedicine appointment time, a member of staff should confirm the patient has successfully connected and they may also perform a review of requisite materials and information for the visit. In many respects, one should conduct the visit in the same sequence as they find productive during their in-person clinics where admin or front desk staff can ensure they have the patient details for billing and follow-up, nursing staff can review the patient's history, medications, allergies, and collect or review any measurement from connected devices. Such processes will often be familiar to your patients and can act to make the visit seem more familiar, and patients will be less apprehensive about things going wrong when they're talking to their physician.

Optimize your medical record system

The documentation requirements for a telehealth service are the same as for a face-to-face encounter. The information of the visit, the history, review of systems, notes on the consultation, or any information used to make a medical decision about the patient should all be documented. Whether or not you utilize an electronic health record, having a system in place where each of the staff can review and record details as part of their workflow and allow the chart to be available for the next user in the workflow is something that can and should be planned for. Adopting and using a separate telehealth-only electronic notes system, is not something which I currently can recommend or see particular value in. If you are relying upon telehealth devices or measurements, some may come with their own platform or cloud-based interface; it is wise to have a system in place to document these as they are reviewed, and store a copy of the results directly in your (electronic) medical record.

Depending on the context of the care provided, it may also be important to prepare workflows to ensure adequate documentation for reimbursement. For example, some health insurers require documentation of a certain minimal set of data before they will reimburse providers. The following list includes examples of each of these, along with sample text one might find helpful:

- Patient consent should be documented. Very often providers must document confirmation that the patient agrees to receive services via telehealth—even verbal consent, but it must be documented.
- The method of telehealth (for example: Consultation was performed via secure two-way interactive video connection over _____ [insert video platform name here] ___).
- Provider location. (For example—The provider was located at __ [clinic, city, state] __).
- Patient location and disposition. (For example—The patient was located at __ [city, state]__).
- List all other clinical participants, roles, and actions. (For example— Consultation with ___patient__, with ____RN___, who reviewed the patient's medical history, medications, and allergies, and obtained vitals and patient weight; and _____MD___ who conducted the physical examination and consultation with ___ [the patient]__).

- The amount of time spent discussing the medical reason for the consult, and often may require start and finish times if a service was offered. (For example: The consultation including discussion of treatment options lasted 30 minutes. In addition, a 15 minute counseling session on smoking cessation was also provided by ____RN___ and started at 9:15 a.m., and concluded at 9:30 a.m).
- Other documentation requirements are the same as a face-to-face encounter.

Patient and provider investment in hardware

While most practices will have some computer equipment, to begin a telehealth practice, you may need to invest in some additional hardware. This includes desktop computers, laptops, and smartphones. For telehealth visits, and particularly if existing desktop computers are older, you may need external webcams or speakers. While approximately 86% of the population of the European Union have a smart phone, ~85% in the United States of America, and ~75%–80% in Australia and South Korea, one should not assume their patients will have both a suitable device and a suitable internet connection. While advocating for greater patient access should remain a priority for all who pursue the provision of better and more equitable healthcare, it is now evident that the majority of patients in such nations will already have a suitable device and connection, whether a laptop, tablet, or suitable cellular phone.

Billing and coding integration

Implementing telehealth requires a thorough understanding of eligibility, terminology, and billing. Approval and documentation requirements for telemedicine visits differ by classification, and familiarity is essential for coding and billing compliance. Virtual services include telemedicine visits, virtual check-ins, and e-visits.

Telemedicine visits (aka video visits) allow patients to interact through the necessary elements of both live and interactive audio and video. This can be used for both new and established patients as well as patient consults. The billing and documentation can be considered the same as for in-person visits, and so have the highest revenue potential.

Clinician phone visits are scheduled, telephone (two-way live audio)-based encounters between the patient and provider, and not originating from a related emergency medicine service provided within the previous week, or leading to an emergency medicine service or procedure within the next 24 hours. New and established patients can use this option (as a result of a recent change). These visits are billed according to the time spent in direct telephone contact.

A virtual check-in is a brief, non-face-to-face encounter between a patient and a physician that use digital communication technology. Eligibility requirements for virtual check-ins are less stringent than for telehealth visits, and documentation requirements are also less extensive. It may be a brief telephone check-in call with an established patient between a physician or advanced practice provider to decide whether an office visit or other service is required. These have a minimum duration of 5 min in direct contact. These contrast with a "remote evaluation of recorded video and/or images" submitted by an established patient, and where the visit has not originated from an emergency medical visit within the previous 7 days or lead to an emergency services or other procedure within the next 24 hours.

E-visits contrast further as they are non-face-to-face encounters between a patient and a physician that use asynchronous (not real-time) digital communication technology. E-visits are for established patients who have had an appointment at most within 1 year prior, and the entire consult occurs via a digital platform—like a secure patient chat or the secure patient portals many may be familiar with in electronic health records. E-visits cannot be used to relay results or schedule appointments but can be used for digital evaluation and management.

Information technology support

As with the adoption of any new process, procedure, or technology, there is always a learning curve. While urologists are well accustomed to learning curves from their own professional development as multiproceduralists, a similar learning process can and should be adopted for implementing a telehealth service. Obtaining mentorship and maintaining supports in the form of those more experienced in telehealth systems, whether other colleagues or IT support, is particularly important while practices and physicians navigate their way along the learning curve of telehealth provision.

Audiovisual platforms

For those at institutions, many will already have agreements in place with a video conferencing or teleconsult service, and some may already have integrated these services to their electronic medical record (EMR). There are a number of online providers who have Health Insurance Portability and Accountability Act (HIPAA) and General Data Protection Regulation compliant services for medical video consultations. Important considerations when choosing a provider include network reliability, ease of use for patients, and those providers that do not require patients to have an account. Some widely used platforms are Doxy.me and Doximity.com, which offer features such as a text message sent to the patient's smartphone device, and a single link will permit them to start a video chat with their provider. In the United States, there are temporary waivers for HIPAA, which permits the use of other noncompliant platforms, but one doesn't need to transmit confidential patient information or leak even more metadata to such tech behemoths, so one should not.

Patient and caregiver participation

It is imperative that regardless of the modality used to interact with patients, healthcare remains patient-focused. While many urologists might spend a great deal of time and resources focusing on their own ability to provide this service to patients, one should consider better ways to perform a teleconsult and enable better uptake for certain patients—particularly those who may require in-home support or the help of caregivers to facilitate their visit, whether in person or online. There is a need to consider your "webside" manner as well as your bedside manner.

Deciding what services to offer

A useful metaphor for deciding what services to offer, is considering how urology trainees acquire surgical and other skills. Start with relatively simple procedures which help gain confidence in fundamental principles, including developing confidence and competence in using tools, and troubleshooting when things don't work as they should.

As confidence is gained, one can gradually, and in a step-wise fashion, introduce more complex procedures to their telehealth practice. A sample framework of services is listed below. This should be considered a general list, but individual practices may weigh technical, workflow, and change management differently and so these may be different for your practice.

Providing telehealth (audio and video) visits to patients for routine follow-up of noncomplex conditions.

- Requires relatively little new hardware
- Many are already familiar with these technologies
- Patient and physician already have an established relationship

Incorporate e-prescribing to your care

- Integrating the practice into your workflow and documenting and billing as appropriate
- Many patients are familiar with the concept of prescriptions being "called in" to a pharmacy for them, but some may require additional prompts or follow-up to make sure they remember to collect the prescription and start therapy

Telehealth visits to new patients, where the presenting complaint is unlikely to be complex or complicated.

- This may require changes to practice workflow, particularly administrative work, collecting new patient's details, and obtaining various consents.
- Guiding staff and ensuring buy in may take some time as many are often reluctant to adopt change.
- It is also important to remember that not every visit is suitable for telehealth care; this step will allow for providers to gain confidence in knowing when to convert a televisit, to an in-person visit, and all of the steps, from counseling the patient to scheduling and coordinating with other staff, to arrange for an in-person visit.

Incorporate remote patient monitoring of chronic conditions for patients who have had a relatively stable condition, or where the course of their disease has been relatively predictable.

- Introducing new hardware to patients and incorporating hardware, software, and other IT integrations that may be required are often best performed in the context of caring for patients with relatively stable and chronic illnesses first.
- This will also likely introduce more workflow complexity, and initially may require additional time to review information either before or during the visit.
- Increased administrative complexity and introducing staff to new billing procedures/billing using codes not used before may be required.

Incorporate remote and digital diagnostic procedures to your care.

- Introducing new technology, but where the provider and patient depend on a reliable and consistent result, and for it to be provided immediately and in realtime during the consult, introduces all sorts of complexity. It is best added after similar issues have been overcome by all members of the medical practice.
- Staff will be becoming more familiar with changing and new administrative and billing procedures, as well as documentation requirements

Offer telehealth visits to all patients including those requiring coordination of multiple diagnostic procedures and investigations, and which may require multidisciplinary input.

- Trying to provide technical support for your own office, the patient and colleagues can be overwhelming. Complexity can be reduced by reducing the odds of either your practice or your patient having an insurmountable technical issue during such consults. This can be achieved following a gradual and stepwise introduction of the tools and technologies to all stakeholders in healthcare.

Bibliography

Chu, S., Boxer, R., Madison, P., Kleinman, L., Skolarus, T., Altman, L., … Shelton, J. (2015). Veterans affairs telemedicine: Bringing urologic care to remote clinics. *Urology, 86*(2), 255–260. https://doi.org/10.1016/j.urology.2015.04.038

Smith, W. R., Atala, A. J., Terlecki, R. P., Kelly, E. E., & Matthews, C. A. (2020). Implementation guide for rapid integration of an outpatient telemedicine program during the COVID-19 pandemic. *Journal of the American College of Surgeons, 231*(2), 216–222 e212. https://doi.org/10.1016/j.jamcollsurg.2020.04.030

Infrastructure and security in telehealth

Introduction

The term infrastructure is derived from the Latin word "structura", meaning—a fitting together, or to pile/assemble together, and "*infra*" meaning on the underside/beneath; this chapter will focus on understanding the elements that are piled together underneath the telehealth system, so that the practitioner can understand, "what is beneath the hood." These are not necessarily the brick-and-mortar components, but predominantly the elemental components of the system. The system is not just your office, or your local network, or even your country, it is indeed much larger than that. For example, the components comprising the infrastructure which are in everyday use, include elements which are extraplanetary and reside in outer space.

The infrastructure required in your office may be dictated by a number of factors ranging from regulatory requirements, capital available, right through every link in the network, and may even be influenced by bottlenecks in bandwidth; if your patients are unlikely to have access to high-speed broadband with low contention ratios, then it is tempting to design your infrastructure around this bottleneck. There is little need to have high-definition 4k video equipment if your internet service provider is transmitting information over copper telephone wires, or if your patient is unable to receive such high-definition video. However, it seems evident that we will look back at such statements with the sort of adoring condescension and bewildered incomprehension, that a modern adolescent might have for the significance of the spinning jenny. That is to say, there will be a time, and very soon, where affordable access to high-quality, high-speed internet access, will be ubiquitous. Technology is currently available to load balance and match bandwidth as appropriate, so that users do not experience the infuriating spinning wheel, that symbolizes a buffering video. I would actively encourage all in telemedicine, to come to understand the tools they use to deliver care, much in the same way it is important for a surgeon to understand, not only that electrocautery works, but also how it works, so that they can understand how it can be misused, and how the understanding of its function is necessary, so that harm to patients may be avoided.

The infrastructure requirements were alluded to briefly in the first chapter of this book, and some of these components will be discussed in more detail here. There are many ways in which we can interpret infrastructure in the context of telehealth. For a

Telehealth in Urology. https://doi.org/10.1016/B978-0-323-87480-9.00007-5

busy practice, one can and should consider that offering telehealth visits is akin to building an extension to your physical practice. You may find that with considered scheduling, telehealth visits for suitable patients and consultations, do indeed offer the physical space and time for consultation rooms to be used by allied health professionals, and to be prepared properly, while the clinician is occupied with a telehealth visit, and so allow for greater efficiencies within the practice.

One can classify the infrastructure components required in many ways, and using geographic location as a rubric is a useful starting point. Some may read this chapter with more attention to what is local, but again I would stress, that the network is only as strong as the weakest link, only as fast as the slowest interlink, exchange, section of fiber, or roll of copper wire. It is only as robust as the legislation that exists to define its scope and nature, regulation, and protection. I would urge the reader to consider all of the elements. A few of these factors (local and national) will be discussed in more detail, so that the reader can appreciate that while telehealth promises to make access easier, it only does so for those who have access to the devices and services required to conduct a telehealth visit.

Personal and personnel requirements (local factors)

Practitioner demeanor is fundamental to all patient care. Urologists are among the greatest innovators in medical sciences, and have seen and helped lead great change in surgical practice so far this century and last. As a specialty group, many are proud of the nature of the specialty to troubleshoot issues with robots, lasers, endoscopic tools, scopes, and all sorts of digital and analog tools used in practice. The same mentality is required in telehealth. The same openness and cautious evidence-based approach to change is required. Whether that be, adapting new practice procedures and protocols as becomes necessary, evolving to run hybrid clinics, or moving toward sessions which are entirely offered by telehealth. The same dynamism that allows urologists to maintain a diverse skillset from open to minimally invasive surgical skills, from andrology to oncology, fertility to reconstruction, is what is required to adopt telehealth and begin adapting one's practice to incorporate telementoring, telediagnosis tools, and telemonitoring tools.

In much the same way, it is imperative to have a similar culture across one's practice. Having coworkers and colleagues willing and able to incorporate something new and sometimes challenging, is equally as important. Being able to welcome new challenges, and using telepresence and digital tools to help improve patient care, is a significant change, and time and training required for staff to gain confidence in their use, will pay dividends and give greater confidence to patients who deserve competent and confident care. Technology can and should make our lives better and safer. But its use often requires careful and considered planning to ensure that everything from the cameras, microphones, digital records, digital patient and practice schedules, and digital payment systems are maintained, secured, and properly used. In many ways, these are reflected by the culture of the healthcare organisation or urology practice, and take time to develop.

Lobbying for better access (national/state-level factors)

While many advocates of telehealth will espouse, the platform allows greater access to better health. However, this is only the case for those who are willing and able to use such portals, and perhaps more critically, for those that can afford and have access to appropriate devices and providers of cellular and internet access. One should not assume that because someone lives in a large metropolitan area or a "developed" nation, that they have access to adequate broadband internet. The average connection speeds in 2020 were ~ 42Mbits/s in the United States and 103Mbits/s in the European Union (EU). While these are adequate for videoconferencing and a video consult, remember that gigabit connections were expanding in these regions before 2020, and that these outliers will buoy those average values.

While access to healthcare has long been a priority policy point for healthcare advocates, access to reliable, high-speed internet and suitable devices to conduct telehealth visits, becomes synonymous with access, in a world where telehealth becomes the norm. While some may see this as complicating the issue of access to healthcare, it should be remembered that health access was always complicated, and that with these few infrastructure pieces in place, access to the whole array of health services can become a lot simpler. Consider a patient who needs to see their general practitioner, ophthalmologist, audiologist, podiatrist, occupational therapist, and physiotherapist. On top of the complexity to manage the scheduling, the patient is encumbered with the logistics of getting from one department to the next on time, and from one building to the other, and often these are geographically dispersed practice locations. If one considers that $\sim 10\%$ of the US population >18 years of age report some mobility difficulty, and according to the CDC, 26% of adults in the United States of America report some type of disability, one now can appreciate that attending medical visits in person can quickly become a near full-time occupation for those who need multidisciplinary medical care (Iezzoni et al., 2001). It is therefore important for healthcare workers and practitioners to lobby and promote for better access for patients, and also for easier access for physicians to practice telehealth, to offer alternative routes to access care, and unencumber this significant proportion of the patient population. That is not to say there should be no regulation, and as with most things in the age of the internet, consumers and healthcare providers require protections from those who would seek to exploit such systems. It should also be remembered that while everyone should have access to adequate and sufficient healthcare, that healthcare is not a consumer product. "Productified" health is not healthcare, and many consider it exploitative of patients and physicians and to the detriment of societal well being.

Wireless communication infrastructure

Mobile telecommunications technology continues to evolve, and now even, the term "3G" seems archaic. Research and development of 3G technology started in the

1980s, and by 1999, the International Telecommunication Union (ITU) approved 5 radio interfaces for the standard, with the frequency spectrum ranging from 400 MHz to 3 GHz. 3G is the short form for "third generation" and is used to describe a mobile phone standard. 3G networks enable you to make voice calls and send texts as well as access the internet—giving you the ability to browse the web, check email, and download content at speeds of up to 7.2 Mbps, (although the standard defined by the ITU does not include this). A statement by the ITU did provide some guidance on data transfer speeds, where a minimum data transmission rate of 2 Mbits per second for stationary or walking users, and 348kbits per second in a moving vehicle are required. In practice, 3G download speeds depend on the underlying equipment the providers ultimately installed, where up to 384kbits/s is possible for Universal Mobile Telecommunications System (UMTS); High Speed Packet Access (HSPA), and HSPA+ could potentially provide download speeds of up to 7.2Mbits/s and 21.1Mbits/s, respectively.

Fourth generation (4G) and 4G Long-Term Evolution (LTE) launched circa 2010 and offered not just faster data transfer speeds but also upgraded security. Throughout the evolution of wireless technology, the push to increase bandwidth and transmission speeds has been a catalyst for creating new wireless technology standards. With this we have seen fifth generation (5G) networks become more widespread in the last 3 years (see Table 4.1). 4G uses lower frequency bands (with longer wavelengths) below 1 GHz, while 5G uses higher frequencies (and lower wavelengths), and so has greater challenges with signal propagation. Therefore, the distance 5G radio waves can travel is much more limited than 4G, particularly in densely populated areas.

Both 4G and 5G utilize a public key infrastructure (PKI) system, which is a method of establishing the identity of devices using cryptographic keys. This is an important point, but first one must appreciate how PKI works: public key and private key are created by a certification authority (CA) for each device. The private key should only ever be known to the device that needs an identity, and the public key can be distributed to any part that needs to encrypt messages to the device, for example, the cell phone service provider. The CA that creates these keys is

Table 4.1 Speeds attainable by wireless communication devices by "generation."

Year	Generation (G)	Data transmission capability
1980s	1G	Voice only
1990s	2G	+SMS text messages
2000s	3G	1–2Mbits/s
2010s	4G	2–100Mbits/s
	4G LTE	10–200Mbits/s
2019	5G	200–634Mbits/s

trusted by all devices in the chain that need to check the validity of the certificates. When a device needs to connect, it will present a message signed by its private key to the authorization system. The authorization system will validate the message by decrypting it with the public key that corresponds to the private key of the device. The system will also verify that the public key it used was created by the trusted CA, so it knows the certificates are valid. If all these checks pass, the system will be able to confirm the identity of the device. With 4G devices, the keys for the cryptographic system are placed permanently on the SIM card, (the universal subscriber identity module card). These are permanent keys, and so this complicates security, as if these are disclosed or somehow compromised, keys cannot be reissued without physically changing the SIM card. According to research by Ericsson (https://www.ericsson.com/en/reports-and-papers/mobility-report/dataforecasts), the Swedish networking and telecoms company, that as of June 2022, there are 5.34 billion unique mobile phone users (>2/3rds of the world's population), and more impressive is the number of connections from Internet of Things (IoT); as of 2022, there were 14.6 billion IoT connections worldwide, and most of these are using 4G or older technologies. This places the significance of a data breach on cryptographic keys in context, and one should consider just how complex, labor intensive, and challenging it would be if even a small percentage of keys required replacing.

5G networks offer a potential security upgrade as its rollout and adoption offers the opportunity for new security protocols. However promising this sounds, this is just one area of vulnerability in such networks, and a number of "security" firms who offer cellular device hacking tools for sale such as NSO (who sell Pegasus spyware) and QuaDream (who sell REIGN) can take control of smartphones and bypass all of these cryptographic protocols entirely. It should be noted that the software products on sale from such firms can take control of the device without the user knowing, and can therefore take control of any connected device that may receive commands from that smartphone. But it also paints a worrying picture where other smart devices, whether insulin pumps or inhalers, can be interfered with.

What urologists should know about spectrum allocation?

While some of this may seem like historical miscellany, it is important to understand the context of spectrum allocation for a number of reasons. First, the bandwidths and frequencies are not unlimited. Many who listened to terrestrial radio are familiar with two radio stations of a similar frequency, interfering with each other, this is known as tropospheric ducting. This is when signals bleed into one another. To avoid this, and because bandwidths are finite, allocation of bandwidth must be respected and may require regulation to avoid interference. In the early part of the 21st century, governments in the EU and United States allocated the finite frequency spectrum, following an auction. In Europe, over 20 years ago, over $100 billion was collectively paid for these frequency spectrum allocations by private industry.

The allocations in the United States are particularly notable, as the entire spectrum was not auctioned. (This is likely the case elsewhere also; however, more information is available on the United States). A significant part of the spectrum was allocated to the US Department of Defense. With growing saturation of commercially available bandwidths, lobbyists have pushed for the Department of Defense to cede or share some of their bandwidths to private industry. Separately there have been discussions about cooperation of the Department of Defense sharing some bandwidth for medical applications, as for a period of time, only they had sufficient bandwidth available, which was reliable enough, secure enough, and with low enough latency to facilitate entirely remote robotic-assisted surgery.

In 2020, the US Department of Defense published an Electromagnetic Spectrum Superiority Strategy. This is a plan to ensure that the United States maintains its military advantages in the electromagnetic spectrum. The strategy has three main goals: to control the electromagnetic spectrum, to deny adversaries the ability to use the electromagnetic spectrum, and to protect the United States from electromagnetic threats. The strategy also includes a number of initiatives to improve the United States' ability to operate in the electromagnetic spectrum, including developing new technologies and improving training and education. What is similar for defense, as it is for healthcare, is that nearly every form of communication used today in hospitals and by healthcare workers is wireless and leverages the electromagnetic spectrum. The electromagnetic spectrum encompasses all possible frequencies of electromagnetic radiation, from low-frequency radio waves to high-frequency gamma rays. While frequencies above 300 GHz include infrared light, visible light, ultraviolet light, and X-rays, frequencies at 300 GHz and below are used to transmit information for cell phones, television, radio, satellite communications, Global Positioning Systems, Bluetooth communication as well as radio frequency identification chips, commonly used on ID badges, for swipe cards to access buildings and to unlock cars and devices.

For many of the same reasons that the US Department of Defense sees it as a strategic imperative that they have unrestrained, unfettered, and exclusive access to an entire block of the spectrum, one can see the importance for healthcare to have a similar level of access. Commercial advancements proliferating wireless devices and services will continue to erode the capacity for healthcare to utilize the finite resource that is the electromagnetic spectrum. As the airwaves become saturated, how can access be equitably distributed? If healthcare delivery (via telehealth and wearable devices and sensors) will rely upon access to the available electromagnetic spectrum, should the provision of a pacemaker come with a monthly plan? Will those providing connected health have to compete with discretionary consumer spending categories from "connected accessories" from car manufacturers, to cell phone and computer companies, television networks, and retail, social media, and search behemoths, for the limited space available?

The future proliferation of electromagnetic spectrum-dependent systems in health will include almost all elements of healthcare, from diagnosis, monitoring, population health surveillance to treatment and rehabilitation. It is incumbent upon those planning for future health systems, public health officials, healthcare systems, and all stakeholders in healthcare, to advocate and ensure sustained future and equitable access for healthcare systems. And much like the practice of evidence-based medicine, it is also imperative that those in healthcare understand the risks and benefits, the consequences of its use, and any potential adverse effects, arising from the use of such products, devices and services. We will discuss this in a separate section later in this chapter.

What urologists currently use the electromagnetic spectrum for in everyday practice?

Different parts of the spectrum serve different health purposes. X-rays have been in routine use in medical care for over a century, being used 6 months after Roentgen's discovery to identify bullets in wounded soldiers. Other segments of the spectrum are not as often considered for their utility in medicine, yet those uses are no less essential for healthcare to function. For example, radio waves are still utilized by many health systems using pager systems. They still have advantages over cell-phones as they can travel (relatively) long distances and pass through solid objects like buildings and trees, and even receive messages in hospital basements and through lead-lined walls in radiology departments. Microwaves have higher data rates than radio waves and are often used for satellite communications, internet access, and other communications. Microwave energy has also been used in medical treatments for over 40 years, and there are a number of applications in use including tissue ablation, and also in applications such as sterilization. Infrared is of course closely associated with heat sources, and is widely applied in noncontact thermometers, and in screening equipment in waiting rooms and entrances to facilities. Infrared light can be used to help treat conditions such as pain and is widely used as part of rehabilitation therapy, and by others to aid in wound and tissue healing. It has also been adopted in some surgical systems to help visualize blood vessels and tissue perfusion, with the ability to discern relative levels of perfusion and blood flow, and so has applications from disciplines as varied as reconstructive surgery and cancer surgery, to stroke care and vascular surgery. Gamma rays are also familiar to the practicing urologist, as many will have had questions from patients on the "gamma-knife" surgeries performed by radiation oncology colleagues. Gamma rays have the shortest wavelengths and greatest energy on the electromagnetic spectrum, and owing to their properties, are widely used in tissue destruction (or radiation therapy). Gamma rays when administered in sufficient doses are also lethal to prions, viruses, bacteria, and other microorganisms, and so are also used to sterilize medical equipment. Gamma rays are also used in nuclear medical imaging techniques such as positron emission tomography (PET) imaging.

Risks of electromagnetic radiation to patients—long-term exposure to different parts of the spectrum

This section briefly addresses what is known of the health effects of exposure to electromagnetic radiation, as there is ongoing concern among the general public.

While the effects of exposure to gamma rays, X-rays, ultraviolet, visible light, and infrared light and their role in disease and medical applications are better understood, those of longer wavelengths are usually the subject of public concern. In response to these concerns, the International EMF Project was launched. It is a research initiative of the World Health Organization (WHO). The project was established in 1996 in response to public concern about possible health effects of exposure to electromagnetic fields (EMFs). The project's objective is to assess the scientific evidence of possible health effects of EMF in the frequency range from 0 to 300 GHz—in other words, as far along the spectrum as microwaves (Fig. 4.1).

Some members of the public have attributed a diffuse collection of symptoms to exposure to EMFs at home. Symptoms reported include headache, anxiety, depression, nausea, fatigue, and loss of libido. According to a WHO report, scientific evidence to date does not support a link between these symptoms and exposure to EMFs. At least some of these health problems may be caused by noise or other environmental factors, or by the fear associated with the presence of new technologies.

More specifically with regards to the risk of cancer, the evidence for EMFs having an effect on cancer remains highly controversial. The results to date contain many inconsistencies, but no large increases in risk have been found for any cancer in children or adults. A number of epidemiological studies indicate a slight increase in the risk of childhood leukemia with exposure to household radiofrequency magnetic fields. However, research work to date has generally not concluded that these results indicate a causal relationship between field exposure and disease, (as opposed to artifacts, or under-study effects, unrelated to field exposure). This conclusion was reached in part because animal and laboratory studies did not show reproducible effects consistent with the hypothesis that the fields cause or promote cancer. Large-

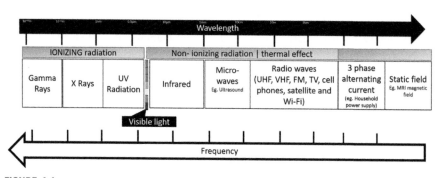

FIGURE 4.1

Frequency versus wavelength across the electromagnetic spectrum. Consider the wide variety of applications in urology which use technologies predicated upon developments from various parts of the electromagnetic spectrum, from shockwave lithotripsy to lasers used for photovaporization and from gamma rays and the cyber knife to MRI and ultrasound fusion biopsy procedures.

scale studies are currently underway in several countries, and may help resolve this controversy.

Also of interest to urologists, are studies characterizing the impact of frequencies commonly used by cellular devices on male fertility. There is no definitive answer to this question as the research is inconclusive. Some studies suggest that there may be a negative impact of mobile phone use on male fertility, while other studies find no significant effect. In general, studies to date have been of poor quality, and provide little evidence. There have also been interesting studies demonstrating effects on DNA integrity after magnetic resonance imaging, which do not help isolate which component of the EMF may be causing the effect. It should be pointed out that studies examining this have demonstrated that the effects on DNA are different in character to those induced by ionizing radiation, and are more similar to those induced by endogenous processes, and so are not necessarily a sinister process (Hill et al., 2016; Scientific Committee on Emerging and Newly Identified Health Risks, 2015).

What urologists should know about spectrum vulnerability?

The aim of discussing vulnerabilities in systems utilizing the EMS, is not to discourage the use of technologies which utilize wireless protocols, but rather the opposite. Urologists themselves and the wider healthcare community must be encouraged to appreciate the potential vulnerability and the importance of not just securing your own local network but also the larger network, which patients rely upon. Urologists must adopt and advocate for practices to protect patients from such system vulnerabilities.

If healthcare uses, and continues to rely upon commercial providers and the allocated commercial spectrum, it will inevitably fall victim to attacks that may not have intended to target health provision. An electronic or cyberattack targeting a communications firm will affect all those who use the service, including hospitals and patients. The nature of a commercial system is such that end nodes or devices used by users, are most vulnerable to attack by an ever-growing number of malware and spyware threats; even if data are encrypted in transit, such tools are unaffected as the data are unencrypted on the end device so it can be interpreted by the user.

Whatever of a visit failing to happen due to lack of service, consider how a malicious actor could impact healthcare provision. This is a reality that many already have firsthand experience of. The world has witnessed multiple ransomware attacks specifically focused at healthcare providers.

Securing a segment of the relevant spectrum for healthcare applications is essential for safe and effective supply of healthcare, which increasingly relies on this fundamental technology. Privacy breaches have always been a concern in healthcare, even prior to the era of electronic health records. The growth of interconnected health on commercial systems, using commercial networks, connected to a worldwide user base of over 5 billion people, means the possibility of remote access is anything but remote. In times past, paper records were kept in hospitals and only accessible by physical access. Add to this the possibility that data theft will go unnoticed, and that there is access to a more comprehensive medical record, and the significance of this threat is better appreciated.

Security for telehealth

What urologists should know about cybersecurity?

Healthcare is inextricably linked with technology now. There are currently 10–15 connected devices per bed in US hospitals (Coventry & Branley, 2018). As mentioned earlier, this greater connectivity is not just in hospitals. Connected devices provide effective ways to care for patients, especially those with chronic conditions. This offers myriad ways to connect to medical devices. The problem is compounded because devices are often easily accessible, increasing the likelihood of someone with malicious intent, finding them. A single device can provide a potential entry point to larger hospital networks, bypassing firewalls and any rudimentary security steps that are taken. As healthcare systems are among the least prepared for cybersecurity, the lag between when an attack occurs and when the breach is discovered is likely longer than anyone would care to admit, and this further increases vulnerability. Whatever about specific health devices that are made for a specific purpose, many patients like to use their connected device to sync with their smartphone, and more still use their smartphone to access their medical records, increasing the challenge of protecting systems.

The use of legacy systems is widespread in medicine, to the extent that one wonders is it organizational complacency, or absolute ignorance of technology, that allows their continued use. One great example is that of the now infamous "WannaCry" attack of 2017. It was the largest ransomware attack in the world at the time, and it paralyzed the UK's National Health System (NHS) (among many others). To place this in context, the NHS has over 1.5 million patient interactions every 24 hours. What is most remarkable about this attack is that the vulnerability which it exploited was identified and patched by Microsoft by mid-March 2017. More than 2 months later, the NHS was affected because they were using Windows XP as an operating system. The issue being that Windows XP had no longer been supported for security updates since April 2014—3 years before. In early 2014, analysts and technology experts including those at cybersecurity firm Sophos were quoted as noting a steady supply in vulnerabilities to the Windows XP operating system; vulnerabilities that were continuously appearing over a period of 12 years. Despite this, many firms, and not just the NHS, were blind to their need to update their systems software. Furthermore, technology researchers in 2014 knew of exploits which had not been used widely at the time, and predicted that attackers would wait until after Microsoft discontinued support to utilize them, which is of course exactly what transpired.

The cost of an average healthcare breach in 2021 was $9.4 million in the USA

This figure comes from an International Business Machines report, but pales in comparison to larger breaches and the individual impact on patients and providers. Most of these attacks are not even as sophisticated as the North Korean citizens who the US and UK governments have accused of being behind the WannaCry attack. Most of the attacks affecting US institutions in 2021 were simple, and demonstrate complacency on the part of healthcare systems.

The sheer number of targets, the operational sluggishness, and the high ransom prices paid, among other factors, make it likely that healthcare will remain a prime target for such attacks for the foreseeable future. From recent attacks, the pattern is that of attackers attempting to either disrupt operations, or interfere with data in some way.

You're not as prepared as you think you are, and the data you have are more valuable than you think it is: the Conti attack on the HSE

If a hospital can't access its records, or its ability to serve patients is compromised, lives are affected and people can die. An example of such an attack is that on the Irish Health Service Executive (HSE). On May 14, 2021, the cyberattack infiltrated the information technology (IT) systems of the HSE, and in response to this, the HSE elected to shut down its IT systems, and disconnect the National Healthcare Network from the internet. It is the most significant cyberattack on an Irish State agency, and is cited as the largest known attack against a health service computer system in history. To add further context to the degree of disruption, is the timing of this attack, which was when the Irish Health Service, (like those elsewhere around the globe), was struggling with the COVID-19 pandemic. It took more than 4 months to recover from the attack, and despite assurances at the time, it is believed much of the stolen information is available, and is being used by attackers for further exploits. It is known that over 700 GB of unencrypted data, including protected health information was stolen. It should also be noted that in 2021, this health service located in Europe and subject to all the same privacy laws as corporations and entities in the EU, saw it as acceptable to have unencrypted data on their systems; a beginner step in data security. Similar to the WannaCry attack, there was advance notice that such an event could happen. Over a year prior, Interpol had issued a public statement that healthcare institutions were being targeted and urged all such institutions to improve security and procedures to mitigate risk and damage (https://www.interpol.int/en/News-and-Events/News/2020/Cybercriminals-targeting-critical-healthcare-institutions-with-ransomware). Again, a similar pattern of slow reaction time on behalf of the compromised system, is evident. According to an independent report conducted on behalf of the HSE, it is believed that the initial infection of the first work station, occurred on March 18, 2021, almost 2 months before the HSE servers were compromised for the first time. The infection with the ransomware occurred a week after this, and 4 days after multiple hospitals had reported malicious activity on computers within their networks. The day before the attacker executed the ransomware (Conti), the vendor providing Antivirus Security to the HSE emailed the HSE security operations team to highlight outstanding and unhandled threat events. The report highlighted that the HSE did not have a single responsible party for cybersecurity at the time of the incident in 2021.

Conti ransomware has been deemed responsible for the attack, which targets all versions of Window's operating systems. The origin of the attack was believed to be from Eastern Europe/the Russian Federation, and perpetrated by a group classified as a "ransomware as a service" cybercriminal group. While this may sound sophisticated, there were multiple actions by the attacker that alerted the HSE to their presence far in advance of the attack, and yet no meaningful action was taken. The HSE themselves had no registry of what systems and applications were in use across their network, and the HSE had almost no ability to investigate the attack using its own tooling. The recovery of the information was only possible, because 1 week after the shutdown of the IT systems, a decryption key became available; apparently the attackers relented and provided the key without a ransom. Yet it took more than 4 months for systems to be restored.

Being conscious of cyber security for you and your patients

While some may focus on the gaffs made by the attacker and others on those of the HSE, the report on the incident makes it clear how significant a more sinister attack can be, and provides an important reference point to understand just how vulnerable these systems are, even in relatively small health systems like the HSE, and in technologically advanced countries. Some of the content of the report is speculative, and makes suggestions which are in no way applicable to the HSE attack in Ireland; at the time of the attack, the HSE did not have a complete electronic medical record. Much of the information maintained on IT systems by the HSE was administrative and pertains to outpatient appointment dates and dates of procedures, but it also contains names, addresses, and dates of birth. Had the system allowed for propagation to medical devices, this could have been more devastating for those affected patients. But this was not the case, because the HSE did not at that time connect or maintain networking for patient devices, and as already mentioned, HSE IT were themselves slow to respond, because they did not then know what systems and components actually comprised their system. The disconnect between public perception of what such a system contains, and what it actually contains, still persists, but the relatively archaic assembly of the HSE system in many respects, limited the extent of the leak. This contrasts with the WannaCry attack of the NHS in the United Kingdom, which did not see data exfiltrated from their system, but the attack did have self-propagating capabilities by way of an exploit called EternalBlue, which was reported to have been initially developed by the US National Security Agency and leaked by a hacker group in April 2017, just prior to the NHS attack.

The cost of an attack is enormous, not just financially, but also to patients and communities. Physicians like many other professions are privileged with the provision of patient care, and the custody of each patient's information. With that comes a responsibility, ethical and also legal, to protect that information. The various attacks discussed in this chapter may seem like they were unique, or the mitigation efforts were insufficient, or there were other human faults that ultimately led to failure in preventing these attacks. These attacks though, should act as a wakeup call that all individuals, organizations, corporations that are big and small, are vulnerable to such attacks, and indeed even more sophisticated attacks. All organizations need to continually consider the extent to which they are protected, and how prepared they are to respond. Much the same way that fire drills are mandatory in some jurisdictions, and that all health centers should have, and should practice a major incident response, the same is true for major cyber incidents. Regardless of how extensive one's prevention protocols may be, there should be a clear, well-known, and well-practiced plan to respond during an incident, so that care may continue uninterrupted, and then recover from the incident without an impact on patients, their care, and their privacy.

The possibility for all sorts of exploits and fraud can perhaps be multiplied with the greater adoption of telehealth, and so there is greater need for vigilance and engagement with the cyber security world. For example, there is now widespread access to deepfakes to impersonate video and voice of other people. For those less familiar, deepfakes are computer-generated images, video, and audio, that look and sound realistic enough to trick people into thinking they're real. They are made by using artificial intelligence algorithms to generate new faces or bodies that mimic existing people. This technology could be used to imitate either physician or patient, and its use and abuse will likely impact how telehealth is offered. This is just a mere sampling of technologies available, without mention of those unknown or in development which could be used maliciously and would impact healthcare delivery. This is not to say telehealth is any more or less vulnerable than existing in person care, particularly with a motivated bad actor. Rather that the service when online is accessible to the entire population of the internet, 24/7, and that practitioners of telemedicine cannot and should not be complacent about proper measures to ensure safe practice for their patients and themselves.

Risk mitigation

A number of agencies, organizations, and regulatory bodies have introduced rules and standards to enhance and standardize cybersecurity risk management. These range from nonprofit groups, technology firms, and cybersecurity organizations to government bodies like the Securities Exchange Commission in the United States, who proposed rules in early 2022, that all public companies be subject to reporting of cybersecurity risk management and cybersecurity incidents. Others come from the EU's ENISA agency for Cybersecurity, the National Security Agency in the United States of America, ISO International (who have an ISO27001 standard for cybersecurity), and many more. Given that cybersecurity is never static, and that threats to facilities are ever present in cyberspace, with new exploits ever presenting, these will likely undergo frequent revision, as should one's suite of tools for preventing cyberattacks. Given that these will likely undergo many changes, further resources on this topic are detailed in a later section below, and here general principles will be discussed.

The United States National Institute of Standards and Technology (NIST) at the Department of Commerce, has published a report offering guidelines for Smart Grid

Cybersecurity, (known as NIST-IR 7628). While initially published in 2010, it has to date undergone 1 revision in 2014. It provides guidance on the security risks associated with the use of mobile devices, such as laptops, smartphones, and tablets, in organizational environments. It discusses the potential threats posed by mobile devices, and recommends security controls to mitigate those threats. These were not written specifically for healthcare, but the methods and supporting information help guide risk assessment, and are useful regardless of industry, for identifying and applying appropriate security requirements. Again, the report reiterates that cybersecurity requirements should evolve as technology advances and as threats invariably multiply and diversify, and become more sophisticated (National Institute of Standards and Technology, 2014).

The report is available in 3 volumes and is over 660 pages in length. While it may seem intimidating and unwieldy as the topic often does to clinicians, it is relatively accessible. That being said, there are some elementary principles which are common to most cybersecurity risk mitigation strategies, and while different names may be applied, the principles are similar. These principles can be considered in medical terms as governance and audit, preventative care, diagnosis, and treatment, which forms a useful paradigm for cybersecurity in telehealth:

Governance: Identify existing and future potential security risks and manage them promptly. Much in the same way that one audits as part of clinical governance, the same applies to system and network health.

Preventative care: Implement system-wide controls to reduce security risks. Much like public health measures to make sure everyone remains safe and that ultimately society and everyone in it, is healthier because of it.

Diagnosis: Rapid detection of incursions, and understanding the systemic implications of such an infection or network breach. Identifying an incident is not enough, rapidly reporting and acting upon that information is as important, as can be seen from the examples of attacks on healthcare systems discussed earlier in this chapter.

Treatment: Responding to and recovering from cyber security incidents. Consider closing a wound with shrapnel and debris still inside or only partially treating an infection with appropriate antimicrobials; this not only is detrimental to the individual but also society at large as escape mechanisms and methods to avoid future detection can be developed once inside the system.

The Australian Cyber Security Centre has also published principles, which many may find accessible and useful when considering their own risk mitigation plan (https://www.cyber.gov.au/). They largely follow the same structure by calling them—govern, protect, detect, and respond. These are outlined in the following text box.

The govern principles are:
- A Chief Information Security Officer provides leadership and oversight of cyber security.
- The identity and value of systems, applications, and data are determined and documented.
- The confidentiality, integrity, and availability requirements for systems, applications, and data are determined and documented.
- Security risk management processes are embedded into organizational risk management frameworks.
- Security risks are identified, documented, managed, and accepted both before systems, and applications are authorized for use, and continuously throughout their operational life.

The protect principles are:
- Systems and applications are designed, deployed, maintained, and decommissioned according to their value and their confidentiality, integrity, and availability requirements.
- Systems and applications are delivered and supported by trusted suppliers.
- Systems and applications are configured to reduce their attack surface.
- Systems and applications are administered in a secure and accountable manner.
- Security vulnerabilities in systems and applications are identified and mitigated in a timely manner.
- Only trusted and supported operating systems, applications, and computer code can execute on systems.
- Data are encrypted at rest and in transit between different systems.
- Data communicated between different systems are controlled and inspectable.
- Data, applications, and configuration settings are backed up in a secure and proven manner on a regular basis.
- Only trusted and vetted personnel are granted access to systems, applications, and data repositories.
- Personnel are granted the minimum access to systems, applications, and data repositories required for their duties.
- Multiple methods are used to identify and authenticate personnel to systems, applications, and data repositories.
- Personnel are provided with ongoing cyber security awareness training.
- Physical access to systems, supporting infrastructure and facilities is restricted to authorized personnel.

The detect principles are:
- Event logs are collected and analyzed in a timely manner to detect cyber security events.
- Cyber security events are analyzed in a timely manner to identify cyber security incidents.

The respond principles are:
- Cyber security incidents are reported both internally and externally to relevant bodies in a timely manner.
- Cyber security incidents are contained, eradicated, and recovered from in a timely manner.
- Business continuity and disaster recovery plans are enacted when required.

Other useful resources

The European Union Agency for Cybersecurity (ENISA) has worked to help make Europe "cybersecure" since 2004. ENISA collaborates with the EU, its Member States, the private sector, and European citizens to develop advice and recommendations on best practices in IT safety. It helps EU Member States to implement relevant EU legislation and works to make critical information infrastructures and networks in Europe more resilient. ENISA seeks strengthening existing competences in EU Member States through the development of multinational, pan-EU communities committed to improving network and information security throughout the EU. Since 2019, it has been developing IT security certification schemes. More information on ENISA and its work are available at www.enisa.europa.eu.

The United States National Security Agency have issued guides to improve cybersecurity and general mitigation strategies. It builds upon guidance from the United States NIST at the Department of Commerce. https://media.defense.gov/2019/Jul/16/2002158046/-1/-1/0/CSI-NSAS-TOP10-CYBERSECURITY-MITIGATION-STRATEGIES.PDF.

The Australian Cybersecurity Centre most recently published their information security manual in June 2022, and it is available online at: https://www.cyber.gov.au.

Bibliography

Coventry, L., & Branley, D. (2018). Cybersecurity in healthcare: A narrative review of trends, threats and ways forward. *Maturitas, 113*, 48–52. https://doi.org/10.1016/j.maturitas.2018.04.008

Hill, M. A., O'Neill, P., & McKenna, W. G. (2016). Comments on potential health effects of MRI-induced DNA lesions: Quality is more important to consider than quantity. *European Heart Journal-Cardiovascular Imaging, 17*(11), 1230–1238. https://doi.org/10.1093/ehjci/jew163

Iezzoni, L. I., McCarthy, E. P., Davis, R. B., & Siebens, H. (2001). Mobility difficulties are not only a problem of old age. *Journal of General Internal Medicine, 16*(4), 235–243. https://doi.org/10.1046/j.1525-1497.2001.016004235.x

National Institute of Standards and Technology. (2014). Gaithersburg, Maryland.: NIST.gov. Retrieved from https://nvlpubs.nist.gov/nistpubs/ir/2014/NIST.IR.7628r1.pdf.

Scientific Committee on Emerging and Newly Identified Health Risks. (2015). *Potential health effects of exposure to electromagnetic fields*. EMF.

Patient considerations and leading change for telehealth providers

Introduction

In January 2020, telemedicine represented $\sim 2\%$ of all visits to healthcare providers in the United States. By June 2020, this figure was $\sim 80\%$. This huge leap in adoption was of course spurred on by necessity, as traditional care was impossible, and the entire planet was advised to engage in social distancing, and other risk mitigation efforts, to reduce transmission of the highly contagious respiratory virus that has left more than 6.4 million people dead in the 2 years since a global pandemic was declared. But there is another huge reason for this massive uptick in adoption, without which this would never have happened: patients were happy to engage with providers via this platform.

Physicians and providers know that telemedicine is good for their practice because it is an efficient and convenient way to engage with patients. It can allow them to continue treating and educating those who are unable to come to their clinic. But patients are the ones who decide whether to start or continue using telemedicine. To earn their support, we must address the many reasons why patients may not choose telemedicine. All involved in healthcare can help patients overcome fears and reservations, by providing them with education and by making every telemedicine encounter a good one.

As many healthcare providers may feel intimidated and even overwhelmed with the telehealth process, technical jargon, wearable devices, connection and connectivity issues, so too, do patients. Many physicians and providers should consider that they may also need to adapt to provide not only medical assistance, but also technical assistance, so that their patients can access healthcare.

Helping patients and your practice through organizational change

While the world was presented with a once in a generation moment, which could have catalyzed a transition to telehealth, it is clear that regardless of the opportunity and innovation that exist, much of the world was not literate or equipped to partake.

Telehealth in Urology. https://doi.org/10.1016/B978-0-323-87480-9.00006-3

The factors influencing this are many, but fundamental to all innovation is change. Organizational change requires careful thought and engagement, for as many as 70% of all change programs fail.

In the context of healthcare, patients are central to the process and are key stakeholders. A study conducted by the Harvard Kennedy School's Center for Public Leadership found that there are eight key factors that contribute to successful organizational change:

1. Create a sense of urgency around adopting telehealth

If you want to help bring about change, you need to be bold and communicate the importance of taking action now. And there certainly is an opportunity right now to do that—as a highly virulent, potentially lethal virus, which can be spread by respiratory droplets from an infected individual, continues to infect people. Heightening organizational awareness is required, but also heightened awareness among your patients. Help generate and focus that sense of urgency, and remember that this should always be inspired and reiterated from those in leadership positions.

The author of the work on organization change points out that if you want your organization to succeed, you need to create a sense of urgency around opportunities that are both strategically rational, and emotionally exciting. This will help to keep all stakeholders motivated and focused on the company's goals—whether that be by ridding an organization of complacency, maintaining the sense of urgency, or both. In the early days of implementing something new, or undergoing any change in practices or processes, the forces of resistance to such change are strongest. It is important that the leader driving the change, both maintains a sense of urgency and banishes any complacency that may creep in, similar to approaches one might take in helping a patient to successfully implement changes to their lifestyle which impact upon their medical condition. If the urologist is complacent in their work, and in inspiring and motivating change, so too will their patients be, and often so too are their staff.

2. Develop a guiding coalition or dream team for the implementation of telehealth to your practice

While this is the second point, developing a guiding coalition is to the process of change management, what an intact and functional central and peripheral nervous system is to urinary continence. It should consist of members from across your practice or institution, so that check in staff through to medical assistants and nurses are represented, and if it is a larger organization, ensure that all levels of hierarchy are represented. Ideally the guiding coalition will represent each of the functions and skillsets required, and should contain a few outstanding leaders and managers, as well as those who can be trusted to be advocates of the change process. It should be made clear that all members of this guiding coalition are equal, as internal hierarchy can often slow the transfer of information. As a word of advice, do not be dismayed if at first the dynamics of your guiding coalition are uncomfortable, trust that as you lead your group through the process that most members will revel given this opportunity, and many will surpass your expectations.

3. Define the vision and develop change initiatives to capitalize on adopting telehealth

Be strategic in your implementation. Take the time to design and define a strategy what can be executed quickly and with enough energy to make the vision a reality. It is important that the vision is something everyone on your assembled dream team can articulate and feels invested in, one that they can communicate and see a clear path toward, so that everyone can see the path to success and understands it is achievable.

For example, if the vision was a urology practice with the capabilities to offer every practical outpatient service currently possible, taking the time to segment the steps toward a practice that can offer those services to everyone is sensible. Such a process might start with offering follow-up visits to established patients who have been identified as being more technologically literate by a preliminary survey of your practice. Then progressing to offering the same service to gradually more and more cohorts of your practice, who perhaps are less comfortable with technology. By this juncture though, your own staff will have gained confidence in the system from using it with patients who are more comfortable. Then step by step, you can expand the scope of services to a greater proportion of your practice, but make sure you don't forget step 1—maintain the sense of urgency and don't allow for patients to be excluded from the benefits of telehealth. Always remember, that if you help people not just see a difference, but feel like they are making a difference, you can help provide them, both staff and patients alike, with a greater meaning and purpose, and great things can happen.

4. Engage key stakeholders and "enlist a volunteer army"

A clear, ambitious vision and strategy, communicated effectively by your "dream team" who believe in it, will motivate people to get on board without the cynicism that often greets messages from management. If done right, with creativity and passion, this can become a self-sustaining movement that attracts employees who buy into the ambition, and feel a sense of urgency. Your initial team who set out to guide this mission forward will recruit an army of those who want to contribute to the vision, rather than those who feel they have to. While you build momentum among staff and patients, remember that greater traction and momentum will build. As patients report more positive experiences to staff, and as staff relay that enthusiasm to coworkers and other patients, the progress and sense of fully realizing the benefits of telehealth will feel more and more within reach, and people want to be part of a success. Remember to recognize the efforts of those who are already working toward the vision, keep engaging them and reenergizing them, and they will succeed.

5. Remove barriers and empower all stakeholders

As you, your team, and the larger enlisted volunteer army make progress, barriers and speed bumps will become apparent. Routines that may have been required for in-person care, or simply survived for no apparent good reason, may prevent or delay the adoption of telehealth in your practice. Everybody should be on the watch out for phrases like—"we tried that before, and it didn't work", and "that's not how it's done here," or "they're just not able," which are often accepted as answers, and rarely are, but these are indicators of institutional barriers. Help patients and staff remove these blocks. Technology can work for everyone, not just the few.

Perhaps, there is an information technology (IT) policy that will not allow each end user to install updates to the video conferencing application in use in your practice, or there are firewall settings that don't allow certain connected devices to sync properly. Or maybe some of your patients don't connect on time or have problems connecting, which makes them late for their appointment time. You already have the key components with your team and volunteer army to help find out why, and figuring out how to remove this barrier. Provide them the tools and authority to solve this problem, even if this means changing how you do things.

6. Generate and celebrate short-term wins

Big or small, anything that helps move you and your practice toward implementing telehealth, is a win. It can be actions taken, lessons learned, processes improved, or the installation of some new devices. Celebrate these wins, not just with staff, but with every patient. These wins can provide confirmation that the decisions and actions are actually succeeding and that your team and army are succeeding. Great wins to celebrate include unambiguous, tangible results, which are directly related to implementing telehealth—such as installing webcams on the relevant workstations, completing your trial run of a telehealth visit, completing your first telehealth consult, and eventually completing your first hybrid clinic, with in person and televisits.

If you can't see the wins, this is in itself valuable feedback that something is awry. A committed team guiding the implementation can quickly adapt to modify the decisions and actions it has taken to implement telehealth in the practice. It is imperative that you generate small-term wins early and consistently to keep the vision on track, and to deliver the service successfully.

7. Consolidate gains and produce more change

Early successes and wins will reinvigorate you, your team, and patients. This can be used to help sustain and build momentum. You, your team, and telehealth will gain credibility as a viable solution for all, after these early wins. Don't allow complacency to creep back in. Don't forget each of the steps that brought you here—starting again with urgency, get more people involved, offer services to more patients, and offer more services via telehealth. As you do this, you'll experience more barriers, which you, your team, and your patients can remove in due course. Help accelerate the vision to completion, and don't allow the typical cultural tendencies that lead to increasing resistance to arise.

8. Institutionalize this change culture

It's much the same for managing patients as it is for managing a practice, as it is for managing a large organization; to ensure these new positive behaviors are repeated over the longer term, it is crucial that you define and communicate the connection between those behaviors and the successes experienced. For example, explain to each patient that their urinary symptoms improved because of the lifestyle changes that they successfully made. Or explain to your clinic staff that phone call volume reduced because they posted regular updates to your practice website or social media accounts advertising and reminding patients of your practice hours. Or in the case of your telehealth practice, that by contacting first time telehealth patients in advance to guide them through the process, leads to clinics staying on schedule, and higher patient satisfaction.

This last step is what will help sustain the progress made in the first seven. The old must be replaced by the new, and it is challenging when old ways are often deeply rooted into practice routines and procedures. Your guiding team and your volunteer army must not be a separate faction from the rest of your practice, but they must synchronize with each other, and then merge to become one effective unit with the same mission. Grafting this new unit and new set of practices onto the stem and roots of an older and still effective unit, will become harder if any of the prior 7 steps loses momentum, and key among them is maintaining urgency. Indeed, as regulations ease and people become more comfortable about in-person interactions, and the need to socially distance reduces, one should expect the diehard fans of the old ways to attempt to discard what has been gained and what is new. In some respects, a change initiative is never complete, but it certainly isn't until there is incorporation of telehealth into your day-to-day activities.

Implementation strategy

A successful telehealth implementation strategy is one focused not just on clinical practices but primarily focused on patients to enhance the adoption and sustained use of telehealth tools. Successful implementation strategies improve key implementation outcomes including acceptability, adoption, suitability, feasibility, reliability, cost, penetration, and sustainability (Proctor et al., 2011). The Expert Recommendations for Implementing Change project was a study aiming to refine a published compilation of implementation strategy terms and definitions by systematically gathering input from a variety of stakeholders with expertise in implementation science and clinical practice. They also identified through expert consensus,

73 implementation strategies for clinical innovations, which are a great reference for you and your practice as you move through this process.

Proactive versus reactive technical support for patients

Many are well accustomed to having to contact and access technical support when they have an issue. However, I would propose that when one needs to access technical support for their health, as in a telemedicine consult, they are in no fit state to be left to automated phone trees, and provided a technological barrier rather than a medical solution. Preparing patients for telehealth is therefore of the utmost importance, and it is incumbent upon us all to not only advocate for a better standard of telehealth care for all, but also to help educate patients, improve their telehealth literacy, and reduce the distance between patients and healthcare that maybe inserted by technology.

While it might be tempting to outsource technical support to someone else, a patient's experience of your practice is their experience of your care. It shouldn't be the case that patient care and patient experience be outsourced, or offered for tender where only financial cost is considered. The workflow of a telehealth visit is new not only to patients, but also to the practice and its staff, and often the best teachers are those who have just learned that same thing themselves.

It is also important to remember that not every patient will require the same amount of assistance and attention. Some are more technologically literate than others, and perhaps some designed the systems you are using. When clinicians at Johns Hopkins were adopting to telehealth care provision to the masses amidst the COVID-19 pandemic in 2020, they developed a "video visit technical risk score," which they added to their electronic health record system to identify patients that would require assistance prior to their telehealth visit and added it to display a color-coded column in the schedule template. The score runs on a scale of 0–4, where 0 represents someone who is very likely to have a successful video visit and 4 representing someone with the greatest chance of having an unsuccessful video visit. The group at Johns Hopkins comprised their score based on the following factors:

> Two points for not having an active account in MyChart (an online portal for patients to view their electronic health record).
> One point for not having completed an electronic check in process in the seven days prior to the visit.
> One point for not having had a prior video visit in the past 3 months.

> Or

> One point for having had a telephone visit in the past 3 months and no video visit.

These are simple objective criteria which can be automatically calculated from the electronic medical record, and while there are others that may also predict the success of the subsequent telehealth encounter, these are relatively simple to institute.

The Hopkins group employed central IT support, and their frontline clinical and front desk staff, to proactively reach out to patients in high-risk groups, who would most likely need assistance, and started 7 days prior to the scheduled visit. In their instance, they began by sending an automated text message to patients (automated text messaging systems are described in Chapter 6). They initially sent further reminders three days prior and the day prior to each patient's visit, and only to those that had previously consented to receiving communication via text message. In their pilot study, only 2% of patients (7/384) returned a call to the support team for assistance. In the next phase of their work, they offered a text message or a phone call the day before the scheduled appointment. Using this method, they were able to reach 45% (44/98) of patients the day prior to the scheduled telehealth visit. Using their work, it would suggest that those high risk for an unsuccessful video visit be scheduled so that extra time is provided to setup their video visit on the day. Alternatively, opportunistic interventions to improve their ability to access telehealth should be taken when possible, if they have an in-person encounter for any reason, the opportunity could be taken to help them prepare for a future visit, and a small refresher right before the televisit may be sufficient to ensure a satisfactory and successful telehealth visit is achieved (Hughes et al., 2021).

Engage patients with telemedicine

Helping patients get ready for visits is critically important (Fig. 5.1). Much like any other first impression, a patients' first interaction and impression with your telehealth service matters. Invest the time into ensuring patients are ready for their visit, especially their first telehealth visit.

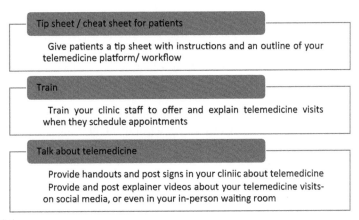

FIGURE 5.1

Tips for improving your patients experience of their telehealth visit.

A useful strategy is to provide patients with a handout to help them understand what lies ahead. For some patients, the use of technology is second nature, and indeed for others, they will encounter specialist care for the first time using telemedicine. But for most existing urology patients, they will have only ever known in person care, and this transition may be a source of stress, discomfort, and even suspicion. Fortunately, there are a wide variety of readymade resources available to help physicians prepare patients—such as those provided in the United States by the Federally funded Telehealth Resource Center https:// telehealthresourcecenter.org. While these are a great resource, practices should take time to use these as a guide and to generate their own resource documents for patients, which help them in preparing for the work flow which your own practice uses. It can be easy to overwhelm a patient with too many handouts and guides, and this would entirely defeat the purpose, and instead add more distress and uncertainty about what lies ahead in the consultation, rather than providing the clarity and guidance that is intended by such a resource.

For some patients, who are less familiar with the technology and technical capabilities of their digital devices, and where resources allow, it is useful to have clinic staff practice visits with first time patients, a process which allows patients to troubleshoot on equipment and logins, remembering to allow permission for their camera to broadcast, and to unmute their microphone, or to reposition their microphone away from a fan blowing directly into it, or other environmental distraction.

It is also really important to remember that when you do create your own bespoke handouts describing what patients can expect at your visits, that it is important to follow the workflow. This helps patients remain at ease and become more comfortable during their visit with you.

Sample information physicians can share with patients to help them understand the value of telemedicine/teleurology

The terms telemedicine, telehealth, teleurology, can conjure up very different images in the minds of different patients. It is worthwhile explaining that these can be as basic as meeting with your patient on the phone or computer, with or without live video, and that many things can be dealt with in such a manner, although not all. Urology is after all a surgical specialty, and physical examination is a crucial component of clinical diagnosis.

As with the introduction of other new or unfamiliar innovations, urologists know that patients often find it useful to hear how telehealth might make sense for them in their situation, and indeed how it has been able to help others. I am reminded of a discussion detailing patients being consented for amongst the first robot-assisted surgeries ever performed in humans; how the patient group being drawn from Detroit, included many who had worked on car assembly lines. Many of them had personally worked with the robot arms, which assembled cars, performing complex maneuvers and lifting heavy components with a precision and consistency that is humbling. The surgeon consenting remarked that this was a group that was able to understand human limitations and see the benefit of having a human work with the assistance of automated processes, robotic arms, and technology. Much in the same way, I know urologists will be able to draw similar parallels with each individual patient that they treat using telehealth tools.

For some, the advert of the convenience of telehealth may not be a feature, as the value of in-person interaction cannot be understated. However, they may not have to find parking, pay a taxi, or have to sit in an unfamiliar waiting room, and that being in their own house by their own bathroom, may be more comfortable for them. For many though, while the process can seem daunting and complex, there are some very simple steps, which are high yield:

- Take time to reassure patients that their health information remains private.
- Address whether their health insurance will pay for their visit.
- Ensure the process is easy to participate in and that you will show them how it works.

Bibliography

Hughes, H. K., Canino, R., Sisson, S. D., & Hasselfield, B. (2021). A simple way to identify patients who need tech support for telemedicine. *Harvard Business Review.* Retrieved from https://hbr.org/2021/08/a-simple-way-to-identify-patients-who-need-tech-support-for-telemedicine.

Proctor, E., Silmere, H., Raghavan, R., Hovmand, P., Aarons, G., Bunger, A., … Hensley, M. (2011). Outcomes for implementation research: Conceptual distinctions, measurement challenges, and research agenda. *Administration and Policy in Mental Health, 38*(2), 65–76. https://doi.org/10.1007/s10488-010-0319-7

What telehealth tools are available for urology?

3

Telehealth tools, conducting a consultation and the ethical practice of telemedicine

Introduction

The basis of the teleconsult is the technology used to speak with and see the patient. There are a number of tools available for this purpose and these are broadly categorized in Fig. 6.1. At the time of writing this book, there are waivers in place due to the COVID-19 pandemic, which allow the use of most video call services, but there will be a time again, when such waivers may not exist, and entirely compliant systems will be required. While many may now employ their smartphone and use the associated video chat functions for telehealth provision, this will not last forever. The use of such systems almost creates a presence in the metaverse for the urologist, who depending on personal preference, may choose to have a separate device, phone number, contracts, and online accounts to separate their telehealth practitioner digital life from their in-person, brick-and-mortar urology practice.

The patient—doctor relationship

Whatever about disrupting healthcare, telehealth has been accused of disrupting the patient—doctor relationship. While telehealth offers to span the geographic distance between patient home and physician office, it could also create distance between patient and doctor, as it could feel impersonal and impact care. Many might be delighted about the newfound promptness with which consultations can be ended in a virtual world, where social norms and etiquette would make a real-world interaction last longer, especially if one of the parties opts to linger longer and share one last anecdote before parting. While some might find these interactions anything from enjoyable to infuriating, they are but one of the many intangibles that form connections between patient and doctor, and promote holistic healing. This relationship between physician and patient can be leveraged to help improve their healthcare, in much the same way physicians use this relationship to help patients improve their health by engaging with new treatments, or to help encourage compliance with care.

Telehealth in Urology. https://doi.org/10.1016/B978-0-323-87480-9.00004-X

Eliminating these unpredictable events can eliminate the authentic nature of individuals in the moment, where that moment, for good or for bad, forms part of the interaction surrounding the medical consultation. Trust, confidentiality, privacy, honesty, and respect are some of the many hallmarks of the patient–doctor relationship. These are formed over time. This is particularly helpful for patients and physicians who have met before a telehealth consultation; as it is very likely a great deal of small talk and nonverbal communication has taken place, and laid the foundation for these hallmarks of the patient-physician relationship, and are essential for good medical care.

Trust is one of the foundational elements of the traditional patient–doctor relationship. A patient's trust is earned by their physician, but influenced by many things, from the tangible—like the office, its cleanliness, its organization, the seats in the waiting room—to the intangible—like the atmosphere in the practice, and how other staff made them feel. If telehealth is offered in a distilled form, as though transactional and feeling hurried, this will affect how a patient perceives their doctor and how they perceive the care they receive. And of course, there are elements which the doctor is not in control of, which will affect how they are perceived by patients—the technology used to power the telehealth consult. Unfamiliar equipment, unreliable internet connections, unsure if their camera is on, or distrusting of whether some connected device is recording every word they say, or that targeted and personalized adverts will soon reflect the contents of what was intended to be a very private discussion with their physician, can contribute to patients distrusting their physician.

Almost 25 years ago, a study of internal medicine consults demonstrated that ∼ 1 in 3 brought up new medical concerns at the end of the visit (White et al., 1997). Another study found that patients were less likely to bring up new concerns when the visit ends with follow-up appointments versus being asked if they have any other concerns (Robinson & Roter, 1999). It is also worth considering that in some contexts, patients prefer to have a family member accompany them to doctors' appointments, and in many face-to-face consults, many will be used to multiple family members, even multiple generations of a family accompanying the patient. While the role of family members as interpreters has been called into question, as they may prioritize their own agenda (Leanza et al., 2010), their roles in providing emotional support, aiding in mobility, and decision-making, is not (Andrades et al., 2013), and consultation models, virtual or in person, should include patients companions or family members whom they wish present for the consultation. Technology should work to enable this, and systems designed and instituted to account for these important factors.

The broad categories of tools for conducting a telehealth consult include virtual phone lines, web-portals, virtual chat platforms and other mobile applications, and will be discussed further below (Fig. 6.1).

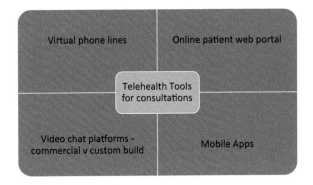

FIGURE 6.1

Categories of telehealth tools available.

Virtual phone

There are companies that provide a "virtual phone" service, which allows one to have an entirely separate HIPAA compliant 2nd line, on their exisiting mobile phone. These services are essentially a virtual 2nd line, with a distinct and separate phone number, but on your primary device. Advantages of this approach include that you do not have to have a second device, that you can set aside "business hours" for your virtual number outside of which you will not be disturbed, and that patients have another option for greater connectivity with their urologist. This could be a disadvantage if this is being used as an additional point for a variety of incoming communications, which could be unfiltered and not triaged. In smaller practices, such a system would be best used in place of other messaging options, rather than in addition to them as it could just add to what is often already a very onerous workload.

Online patient web portal

Many existing electronic medical record (EMR) providers have integrated an online patient web portal to their offerings (Fig. 6.2). These allow patients an alternative to contacting the physician or their office to receive results, or reminders of what was planned, or was discussed at a prior consultation: they are like a digital front desk. There are many versions of these portals from existing EMR providers. It is possible to create one's own custom and bespoke patient web portal, and the optionality and customization, are therefore almost limited by the regulations and the risk tolerance of the provider offering the service. The MyChart offering from EPIC or the Health-eLife from Cerner are two very commonly used web-based patient portals that enable various degrees of interaction and engagement between patients and

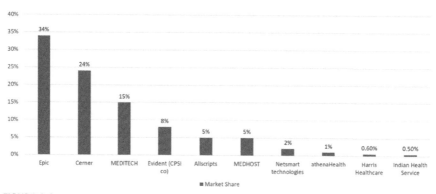

FIGURE 6.2

Market share of inpatient electronic health record systems.

Data from Definitive Healthcare's HospitalView June 2021.

providers. There is plenty of rhetoric extolling the values of patient portals, but in my experience, most patients currently do not derive immense benefit from these as they currently exist. I do believe that there is a generational component to this, both in terms of the understanding of the patients and the providers, but also meaningful interaction is difficult to imbue through existing patient portals that I have experienced. Much of the benefits will come in empowering patients to more meaningfully engage with their own health, but for the majority of people, managing their health is not an everyday reality right now. While I am an advocate and proponent of telehealth, a reality check is required; most people, even those with digital devices designed for these specific purposes, do not know their current blood pressure, the variability in their pulse, or even their respiratory rate and body temperature. When most patients don't know or care to know their most basic vital signs, why would we expect them to fastidiously monitor anything else about their health? There are many important tools and useful components to help improve patient care, and while they must be developed further, we as a profession must help better engage patients with their health from an earlier stage, so that they do care as much about their biological function, as they do about the content of their social media feed, or the release date of content from a subscription streaming service.

Video chat platforms

Face-to-face live communication is now commonplace through proprietary applications, and systems such as Skype, FaceTime, Zoom, and many others, too numerous to list. The days of needing dedicated hardware to provide high-quality audio and video are past, as cell phones have made sophisticated autofocusing cameras and microarray microphones, almost ubiquitously available. For some, video chat—based consultations are telemedicine. This is a not only a case of where unrealistic expectations exist, but also an example of where unaspirational expectations co-exist. Telemedicine is and should be so much more. Telemedicine is not about "giving the customer what they need, as opposed to what they want". Telemedicine and healthcare generally, is not, and should not be about satisfied customers, it is about people, and ensuring they have the best outcome.

Consultations are more than just face-to-face interactions; they often include whole body examination, seeing the patient's surroundings, as well as discussion of results, seeing the results written out, seeing how they change over time or after intervention, and may often involve drawings to help explain a pathology or treatment. And applications like Skype and Zoom offer tools to address many of these issues, such as screen sharing and a whiteboard.

While the choices of available platforms are numerous, there are some important considerations which apply to almost all:

- The provider should use a dedicated space for telehealth consultations, and one that has been optimized for such consults, so that there is no need to reconnect peripherals or devices, or to have to reconfigure the camera or microphone settings. The setting should ideally be tidy and with neutral and calm colors on the walls. Virtual backgrounds are not recommended as they more often act as a distraction, and movements by the physician or practitioner can often result in part of their face being obscured. Positioning of lighting is also important, and be sure that the camera does not point directly at a light source.
- The multimedia nature of a video consult can make it tempting for the provider to look elsewhere while speaking to the patient; this lack of "eye contact", can seem dismissive and portray disinterest. Make a conscious effort to not multi-task while the patient is talking. It is wise to request for patients to disable any backgrounds or camera filters in advance of the consultation, and for them to have chosen a suitable space for the consultation. A video call from a stairwell at their workplace or car is not ideal for most consultations, but of course, these cannot always be avoided.

Conducting a consultation

As practitioners become more accustomed to conducting telehealth visits, they will become aware of factors beyond the obvious, which make telemedicine different to in-person visits. There are distinct skills which the practitioner will develop, some of which are worth mentioning, as such soft skills can often be overlooked. There is a dearth of literature discussing the teaching or conduct of this specialized form of consultation. While some topics may seem less relevant for more experienced clinicians, it is important to review and refresh one's perspective on topics which may seem elementary to your practice. One should employ telemedicine, not in a boot-strapped fashion, but at a standard that meets and exceeds those of best practice for care delivery. These include considering creating new skills; for example, how to perform a clinical assessment and physical exam, when the patient and physician are not in the same room, learning to make the most of new and evolving technologies, and communicating with patients when many of the nonverbal cues are not as easy to appreciate, given the context of the communication. Taking the time to focus and develop these skills may even help to improve one's in-person communication and examination skills, as one refocuses on mastering their craft, albeit delivered by telemedicine. Many of the skills and domains for further development of expertise were recently mapped by, and documented in, a consensus document, which many may find useful as a reference document (Galpin et al., 2021). Some of these are discussed in further detail below (Fig. 6.3).

The ethical practice of telehealth

While there has already been discussion on legal principles relating to the practice of telehealth, in particular on privacy and confidentiality, there is much to consider for the ethical practice of telehealth, as it extends far beyond the concerns of privacy. Telehealth as mentioned earlier in this chapter impacts the patient's relationship with their doctor; it also impacts access, costs, quality, as well as raising issues around health equity, justice, and patient's quality of life. The following will be a brief discussion of how the ethical principles of autonomy, beneficence, nonmaleficence, and justice, can be considered in the context of telehealth provision, and how their providers might consider these in shaping the telehealth practice that they build, and the care that they give via telehealth.

Autonomy

What is new is not always better, and especially while it is new, it may be subverted as much as it may be used for good. Autonomy in telehealth comprises more than obtaining patient consent. Indeed telehealth can both improve and diminish patient autonomy, by increasing the freedom for older persons to remain living in their own homes but also potentially contribute to their isolation and "being made captive' in their own homes (Percival & Hanson, 2016). This backfiring of telehealth was again demonstrated by a UK study that found that while telehealth can improve autonomy for older patients, it may also lead to increased reluctance to leave the home environment for even a small period of time, and reduce independence (Perry et al. 2010).

Others have pointed out that the methods used to collect, store, and manipulate data in telehealth may threaten patients' autonomy if telehealth becomes the primary source of information. A "multipronged approach" that incorporates ethical principles into practice, including regulations, standards, codes of conduct, and codes of ethics, is recommended to reduce this potential risk (Sorell & Draper, 2012).

Knowing when to conduct a telehealth consultation, and knowing when not to

- There are certain situations when a telehealth visit is not appropriate.
- These include when the patient is:
- acutely unwell,
- is in an unstable condition,
- needs an in-person physical examination,
- when in person diagnostic testing is required,
- or when the patient does not consent to a telehealth consultation.

Remote evaluation and care

- Acquire adequate information from a patient during a telehealth encounter to support achieving the desired goals of the encounter.
- Demonstrate how to conduct a remote physical examination. Describe the physical findings that can and cannot be obtained via remote care, and how to collaborate with a telepresenter and the patient to acquire findings.
- Incorporate a patient's observed personal environment into the evaluation, and leverage it to augment the clinical assessment, treatment plan, and therapeutic relationship.
- Incorporate patient-generated data into a clinical assessment and treatment plan, while understanding data limitations and documentation requirements.
- Utilize appropriate telehealth documentation based on modality, health care institution, and practice.

Communicating Effectively

- You may not always see everyone you are speaking with.
- Create rapport, build relationships, and work effectively with
- patients, families, and caregivers;
- referring and collaborating health care providers; and
- remote telehealth support staff (e.g., medical and other health care professionals, and even carers and family members, who are facilitating a remote physical examination).
- Prepare for telehealth sessions, check equipment in advance, wear professional attire, and be conscious that your microphone and camera may always be on, and that patients may still be in the virtual consultation room, even after you think they have left.
- Eye contact, body language and being cognizant for non-verbal queues, are all vital for telehealth communication.

Ethics of telehealth

- Complete telehealth visits in a manner that establishes patient identity, preserves patient privacy, and ensures patient confidentiality.
- Patients have the right to decline care by telehealth in place of in-person care.
- Apply ethical principles, including autonomy, justice, beneficence, and nonmaleficence, to telehealth care.
- Patient access and equity in care; how technology can mitigate and/or exacerbate health inequity and socioeconomic gaps in access to care.
- You shouldn't record your consults.
- Some ethical principles and how they may impact telehealth are discussed in more detail later in this chapter.

FIGURE 6.3

Opportunities for further skill development by physicians to better consider their patients during telehealth consultations, with reference to consensus group statements on telehealth care provision.

Beneficence

Beneficence refers to the ethical principle of doing good or acting in the best interest of the patient. This principle is often applied to healthcare decision-making, and it requires healthcare professionals to consider the potential risks and benefits of any course of treatment before proceeding. In the context of telehealth, beneficence may require clinicians to weigh the risks and benefits of providing care via technology, such as video conferencing, versus in-person.

Telehealth has the potential to help patients by providing assurance, increasing an individual's self-confidence in managing their health, and reducing the dependence on professional caregivers or family (Clark et al., 2010; Eccles, 2010; Iserson, 2000). Improving access, quality of healthcare, and bolstering continuity of care, and expanding the ability for patients to be cared for in familiar surroundings, (like a hospital in the home), rather than as an inpatient, are also beneficent impacts of telehealth (Clark et al., 2010; Eccles, 2010; Iserson, 2000; Keenan et al., 2021).

While many may assume that the actions of healthcare workers pursing better health for their patients to be inherently good, the principal of beneficence should inform, rather than justify other moral principles. One can satisfy this criterion of acting in the best interest of a patient without respecting a patient's autonomy for instance. To be an ethical telehealth practitioner, one should empower their patients to act in their own best interest. Telehealth is a support system for delivery, and caution should be practiced particularly when it is used "as an engineering solution to health" (Gogia et al., 2016).

Nonmaleficence

Nonmaleficence is the ethical principle that states that practitioners should do no harm to their patients. This principle is especially important in the field of telehealth, where practitioners are often not able to see their patients in person, and lean on technology to help provide care.

While telemonitors, not unlike an audio and video monitor used by parents to monitor a newborn, can help promote safety and help provide carers with an extra layer of security and reassurance, the potential for harm is omnipresent with telehealth. Videophones and cameras present in the home, even personal falls alarms, can have the effect of stigmatizing a person, and causing embarrassment or even shame. The devices themselves, wearable or otherwise, can act as a badge of shame, and a reminder to the individual that they are different, whether a burden on others, or in need of help, incapable of being left unsupervised. The devices employed in telehealth themselves can feel alien, and patients feel like they don't understand them and can feel burdened by them (Savenstedt et al., 2006). Indeed, healthcare practitioners may become overburdened by the constant stream of information or distracted by the unfamiliar, and this added complexity and obfuscation of the vital information by novel gadgets, could compromise patient care (Nesher & Jotkowitz, 2011).

Justice

Justice is the principle of fairness and impartiality. Justice applied to telehealth refers to the provision of equitable, affordable, and culturally competent care via distance technologies. It should balance the needs of the individual with those of the wider community, ensuring not to disadvantage one group in favor of another. It is little use to provide a service that nobody can afford for instance, or that aims to eliminate access barriers but ends up creating an economic barrier instead. On a practical point, rural areas often have higher rates of poverty than urban dwellers, and so a technology created to span the distance between rural dwellers and healthcare, may be out of reach for those most in need (Chen et al., 2020; McAreavey & Brown, 2019; Phimister et al., 2000).

Telehealth also professes to improve equity, but for whom? While this may seem paradoxical, consider how telehealth improves equity at the level of individual patients or at the system level (Fleming et al., 2009). There are benefits to be derived from the use of telehealth, which can positively impact on other areas of society and healthcare. However, justifying the expansion of telehealth as improving access for more people by reducing health system costs, ignores the cost to patients who are deprived of social interaction. For many patients a face-to-face consultation with their doctor or other healthcare worker is a much anticipated, and enjoyed interaction, and maybe one of their few occasions to venture out of their home that day.

There also exists a digital divide, and if all practices were to offer only telehealth services, this would be a blatant disregard for the principle of justice. This form of technological determinism must be challenged and caution must be employed. To fully consider the patient in telehealth, one should remember to place the patient firmly in the center of all discussions, so that the quality of healthcare for the patient is not jeopardized by the economic or other interests of private stakeholders. Healthcare provision is about the patient, and healthcare and healthcare providers should work for every patient.

Bibliography

Andrades, M., Kausar, S., & Ambreen, A. (2013). Role and influence of the patient's companion in family medicine consultations: "The patient's perspective". *Journal of Family Medicine and Primary Care, 2*(3), 283−287. https://doi.org/10.4103/2249-4863.120767

Chen, J., Rong, S., & Song, M. (2020). Poverty vulnerability and poverty causes in rural China. *Social Indicators Research, 153*(1), 65−91. https://doi.org/10.1007/s11205-020-02481-x

Clark, P. A., Capuzzi, K., & Harrison, J. (2010). Telemedicine: Medical, legal and ethical perspectives. *Medical Science Monitor, 16*(12), Ra261−272.

Eccles, A. (2010). Ethical considerations around the implementation of telecare technologies. *Journal of Technology in Human Services, 28*(1−2), 44−59. https://doi.org/10.1080/15228831003770759

Fleming, D. A., Edison, K. E., & Pak, H. (2009). Telehealth ethics. *Telemedicine and e-Health, 15*(8), 797−803. https://doi.org/10.1089/tmj.2009.0035

Galpin, K., Sikka, N., King, S. L., Horvath, K. A., Shipman, S. A., & Committee, A. T. A. (2021). Expert consensus: Telehealth skills for health care professionals. *Telemedicine and e-Health, 27*(7), 820−824. https://doi.org/10.1089/tmj.2020.0420

Gogia, S. B., Maeder, A., Mars, M., Hartvigsen, G., Basu, A., & Abbott, P. (2016). Unintended consequences of tele health and their possible solutions. Contribution of the IMIA working group on telehealth. *Yearbook of Medical Informatics, 1*, 41–46. https://doi.org/10.15265/IY-2016-012

Iserson, K. V. (2000). Telemedicine: A proposal for an ethical code. *Cambridge Quarterly of Healthcare Ethics, 9*(3), 404–406. https://doi.org/10.1017/s0963180100003133

Keenan, A. J., Tsourtos, G., & Tieman, J. (2021). The value of applying ethical principles in telehealth practices: Systematic review. *Journal of Medical Internet Research, 23*(3), e25698. https://doi.org/10.2196/25698

Leanza, Y., Boivin, I., & Rosenberg, E. (2010). Interruptions and resistance: A comparison of medical consultations with family and trained interpreters. *Social Science & Medicine, 70*(12), 1888–1895. https://doi.org/10.1016/j.socscimed.2010.02.036

McAreavey, R., & Brown, D. L. (2019). Comparative analysis of rural poverty and inequality in the UK and the US. *Palgrave Communications, 5*(1). https://doi.org/10.1057/s41599-019-0332-8

Nesher, L., & Jotkowitz, A. (2011). Ethical issues in the development of tele-ICUs. *Journal of Medical Ethics, 37*(11), 655–657. https://doi.org/10.1136/jme.2010.040311

Percival, J., & Hanson, J. (2016). Big brother or brave new world? Telecare and its implications for older people's independence and social inclusion. *Critical Social Policy, 26*(4), 888–909. https://doi.org/10.1177/0261018306068480

Perry, J., Beyer, S., Francis, J., & Holmes, P. (2010). *At a glance 24: ethical issues in the use of telecare*. UK. London: Social Care Institute for Excellence. Retrieved from https://www.scie.org.uk/publications/ataglance.

Phimister, E., Upward, R., & Vera-Toscano, E. (2000). The dynamics of low income in rural areas. *Regional Studies, 34*(5), 407–417. https://doi.org/10.1080/00343400050058666

Robinson, J. W., & Roter, D. L. (1999). Psychosocial problem disclosure by primary care patients. *Social Science & Medicine, 48*(10), 1353–1362. https://doi.org/10.1016/s0277-9536(98)00439-0

Savenstedt, S., Sandman, P. O., & Zingmark, K. (2006). The duality in using information and communication technology in elder care. *Journal of Advanced Nursing, 56*(1), 17–25. https://doi.org/10.1111/j.1365-2648.2006.03975.x

Sorell, T., & Draper, H. (2012). Telecare, surveillance, and the welfare state. *The American Journal of Bioethics, 12*(9), 36–44. https://doi.org/10.1080/15265161.2012.699137

White, J. C., Rosson, C., Christensen, J., Hart, R., & Levinson, W. (1997). Wrapping things up: A qualitative analysis of the closing moments of the medical visit. *Patient Education and Counseling, 30*(2), 155–165. https://doi.org/10.1016/s0738-3991(96)00962-7

Remote diagnostics in urology

Introduction

"From inability to let well alone, from too much zeal for the new and contempt for what is old, from putting knowledge before wisdom, science before art and cleverness before common sense, from treating patients as cases and from making the cure of the disease more grievous than the endurance of the same, good Lord deliver us."

(Hutchison, 1998) compiled by Deborah Cassidi in the BMJ in 1998.

Dr Hutchison's words are prescient as healthcare continues to evolve, and it is worth remembering as we discuss telediagnosis. Telediagnosis is a portmanteau of 'tele', derived from the Greek word *telos* meaning distance, and the English word 'diagnosis' meaning just that. (Diagnosis is of course derived from the Greek words *dia* meaning "apart" and *gignōskein* meaning "to know" or "recognize"). Understanding the origin of the terms is indeed appropriate as it provides a framework for what telecommunication must offer, so that a physician can first recognize good health, from disease, and then crucially, discern one pathology from another.

Home-based diagnostics can at present provide targeted services for the care of some urology patients. Advances in technology have been such though, that the only impediment to the practice of entirely remote diagnosis, is a combination of innovators executing what is now entirely possible, and regulators trying to keep pace with the explosion that has occurred, and bracing for the supernova that is surely going to ensue in the area of tele-diagnosis. We find ourselves in a "Wild West" of the World Wide Web, where even legitimate providers of such tools with the best of intentions, have little guidance on what is necessary to adequately protect end users.

Ideal characteristics of medical conditions amenable to telediagnosis

There are many existing tools which will be profiled in this chapter, but the field is ever expanding. In general, the characteristics of diagnostics with the lowest barriers

Telehealth in Urology. https://doi.org/10.1016/B978-0-323-87480-9.00005-1

to entry, in other words, those that are most amenable for rapid if not immediate implementation using current telehealth networks are:

Those that:

- Are amenable to minimally invasive measurement (use sound, vision, or other digital sensors, for external rather than internal and invasive measurement or characterization).
- Require minimal hardware or minimal additional hardware (for example, just use the patient's existing smart phone, or their existing webcam, speakers and microphone, smartwatch, or sleep tracker).
- Do not restrict the patient's life—are already used every day or already exist in the patient's environment—(don't need to install a piece of hardware to their house that occupies physical space).
- Can utilize existing infrastructure that can be secured over existing Wi-Fi, Bluetooth, wired networks, or other telecommunication channels. (Something that isn't going to be interfered with by another nearby device that could affect the reliability of its performance in measuring biomedical characteristics) (Arpaia, Cimmino, De Matteis, Montenero, & Manna, 2012).

At the time of writing this book chapter, the majority of telehealth services, particularly for urological conditions, do not consider the patient as a whole, and in reality, appear to be little more than e-prescribing services, proclaiming to be democratizing healthcare. To the companies who have the legal minimum medical oversight, and employ nurse practitioners or physician extenders to complete screening questionnaires before providing a prescription for medication with little follow-up or patient monitoring, I would assert that the "healthcare" that they profess to be "democratizing" should go the way of the French monarchy circa 1789.

Making a diagnosis is fundamental to the practice of clinical medicine; this is true regardless of whether this practice occurs in-person or via telemedicine. While the practice is complex, some of the core tools of a clinician are rapport building and being able to do so in a short period of time, with a wide range of different individuals, establish the clinical features by history and examination, and interpreting elicited information according to the scientific method (Willis, Beebee, & Lasserson, 2013). Arriving at a diagnosis is not as simple as completing an IPSS or IIEF survey, answering a checklist of questions and calculating a score. The aims of medicine should not just be to diagnose accurately, but holistically. One must formulate an appropriate sequence of investigations, begin appropriate treatment, assess its effectiveness, give an informed prognosis, and make follow-up arrangements. Physicians are not entirely responsible for being seduced by the alures of productified health, as market forces are as real in medicine as they are in commerce. But the medical profession should not become commerce. And while patients many be "consumers" of healthcare, they should not be considered as customers. Many consumers of healthcare have become accustomed to on-demand access, to have their whims satisfied, and I would argue this is a misstep for an effective healthcare system.

The foundations of e-health experience is being conceptualized, designed, and constructed right now. I'd advocate against e-health and telehealth following the path of e-commerce, which seems to be the prevalent model currently in use, where much of the e-health experience is akin to the checkout aisle in grocery stores:

- Much advertising is targeted, and predominant platforms for this are search and social media sites. While this is a powerful tool and capable of much good, these very tools have recently been subverted and used for malicious means to manipulate and even indoctrinate; something which is entirely unacceptable and particularly so when vulnerable groups are being targeted.
- The current e-commerce experience also makes use of prompts to encourage impulse decisions. It has been documented that people make more careful and accurate decisions in the morning time, and make more hasty and inaccurate decisions later in the day (Leone, Fernandez Slezak, Golombek, & Sigman, 2017). The findings of this study are particularly illuminating when cross-referenced with the peak times for e-commerce transactions—between 8 and 9 p.m. at night (Charlton, 2020).

The concern is the "productifying" of healthcare into consumer products. Repurposing the World Health Organization's International Classification of Diseases into a catalog of consumer services to be sold is not useful. While it can be dressed up and presented as noble and worthy, and sold under the guise of improving access, this is clearly a wolf dressed in sheep's clothing.

While some see telehealth as the climate change of medicine (and while in the practice of medicine, such a step change may be welcomed with open arms by many), the value of the patient–physician relationship, with clinical history and clinical examination as core elements, should not be eroded. Clinical history is essential in all cases to generate a logical differential diagnosis and to guide rational investigation and treatment. While in many developed nations, there has already been a steady move away from elements of the clinical exam, as some physical signs pathognomonic of conditions are becoming rarer, and some aspects of clinical examination are being marginalized as novel biomarkers emerge. Clinical examination too is critical to the diagnostic process—recognizing the ill patient and what ills the patient: eliciting signs that cannot be identified with tests and identifying unsuspected problems.

With this in mind, we can approach each of the usual components of the diagnostic process outside of clinical history, to identify what "teletools" are already available to the urologist, and what is possible for teleurology in the early 21st century. The first classification which can be made is whether the diagnostic criteria are subjective or objective (Table 7.1).

Table 7.1 A methodology for classifying diagnostic tools for use in telehealth.

Diagnostic tool is:	Examples
Subjective	Questionnaires
	Diaries
Objective	Clinical specimen
	→ blood, urine, stones, swabs, sweat, saliva
	Electrophysiological parameter
	→ flow rates, urodynamics
	Imaging
	→ ultrasound
	→ advanced imaging
	Procedures
	→ cystoscopy

Symptom diaries, questionnaires, and recording subjective assessments

Symptelligence Medical Informatics (symptelligence.com) have created the "weShare URO" app, a platform for patients with lower urinary tract symptoms (LUTSs). It provides a mobile application where patients can complete validated LUTSs questionnaires and bladder diaries. The platform was examined by some of the cofounders in a 2021 publication following a pilot study of 500 urology referrals, where 45% had among other issues, new LUTSs. The study outlined that the majority of patients were men (M:F = 182:19), and the mean age of patients was 59 years. The mean time from urology referral to initiation of remote or in-office diagnostic and treatment plan, was 7.4 and 7.7 days respectively. This study provides many valuable insights for the field of teleurology: that design and workflow should account for the higher average age of patients who present with LUTSs.

Another application was developed by a research group focusing on pediatric patients. In their prospective study from 2014, they examined a mobile voiding diary for children with voiding dysfunction and compared it with a paper voiding diary. In this study also from the north-east United States, a greater proportion of diaries were completed and had less data gaps in the paper diary than the mobile diary (Johnson, Estrada, Johnson, Nguyen, Rosoklija, et al., 2014) (see Fig. 7.1).

This study is referenced because it is important for a number of reasons: its findings do not suggest superiority of the digital record used over paper-based records. This study was performed at a Children's Hospital in Boston, and families were asked to fill out the voiding diary and excluded those who did not speak English, and those who did not have internet access. The design was also a pre-, post- design, where families had already completed the paper diary, and had already been seen at

a. Home screen   b. Urinary entry screen   c. Bowel movement entry screen

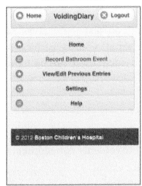 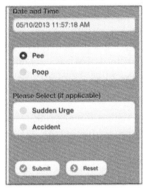 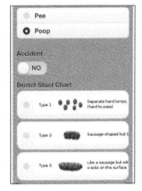

FIGURE 7.1

An example of a pediatric voiding diary mobile application from 2014.

Source Johnson, E. K., Estrada, C. R., Johnson, K. L., Nguyen, H. T., Rosoklija, I., & Nelson, C. P. (2014).
Evaluation of a mobile voiding diary for pediatric patients with voiding dysfunction: a prospective comparative
study. The Journal of Urology, 192(3), 908–913. https://doi.org/10.1016/j.juro.2014.03.099

clinic, and then were asked to repeat the process but this time using a mobile web app of the same questions. This study does not truly assess mobile completion of subjective symptom questionnaires compared to paper versions, and would likely not even be a subjective measure at all, as the parents of children attending the clinic were most likely those repeating the same process, only just doing so on a mobile application the second time.

Blood tests

It is of course possible and acceptable for many to continue to use existing services, where they receive a prescription, or a request is sent to a laboratory testing facility to collect and process specific blood tests. There is no reason why this would not still be useful and particularly for tests, for which identity verification would be wise. Some individuals may try to circumvent a diagnostic process to have medications prescribed inappropriately—such as is reputed to happen with individuals purchasing urine samples from hypogonadic men, only to submit them as their own and to receive testosterone supplements. It is also the case that a significant amount of testosterone supplementation is made without checking a baseline testosterone level (Linhares, Miranda, Cintra, Reges, & Torres, 2021).

This section will also not focus on "point-of-care" (POC) tests (such as Opko's Sangia finger stick prostate-specific antigen [PSA] test), that require the use of specific analyzers and the associated capital outlay. Such analyzers may be in use in a particular clinic, but they are often not practical for "point-of-need" testing, as may be preferred in a truly remote diagnostic setting.

Kits sent by mail

Numerous providers such as letsgetchecked.ie, everlywell.com and www.imaware.com remove the need to attend a testing center. Patients can test themselves at home or wherever they may be. The kits generally need a small volume of blood—$\sim$2–5 drops of blood. For these tests that are currently provided, there are no temperature controls required for the blood sample. The general workflow is:

1. order a blood test kit for delivery
2. collect the sample at home with a finger prick test kit
3. send the sample back (in a prepaid envelope or via a collection service)
4. results are processed in a Clinical Laboratory Improvement Amendments (CLIA)—certified/central laboratory
5. Results reviewed and made available online via a web portal

Lateral flow tests (LFT) for immediate results

Lateral flow immunoassays are a very successful analytical platform to perform rapid on-site detection of target substances. The platform is known by a variety of terms including LFT, immunochromatographic strip test, or rapid diagnostic test. Many people have been exposed to this technology in the form of rapid lateral flow tests for COVID-19, which have become widely available.

It can be considered as a "lab in your hand" for that specific detection of whichever target it has been designed for, and provides a rapid result at the "point of need." And the technology has been applied to a variety of other common scenarios, which can be utilized in the remote care of patients. Their "simple by design" property means no equipment or technical expertise is required; they are very useful in a variety of settings including low-resource environments.

PSA kits

It has been almost two decades since groups proposed, developed, and tested lateral flow tests for PSA—such as the "RapidScreen" test from the University of Rome "Tor Vergata," which generated a positive result for PSA values $\geq$4 ng/mL (Miano et al., 2005). However, at the time of writing, the Food and Drug Administration (FDA) in the United States of America has not yet approved a lateral flow test/lateral flow immunoassay for the detection of PSA for general use.

While such assays with a binary cutoff will not suit every purpose, it is a useful addition to a practice where an initial screening test may be required, so that patients can be reassured while they are still remote from the urology office, and the test is performed in a rapid fashion. The RapidScreen test employs a cutoff of 4 ng/mL, but other kits were developed with alternative cutoff values; in theory, these can be placed at any value above the lower threshold of detection limit, which for some assays is $\sim$1 ng/mL (Bock et al., 2020) when using silica-coated CdSeZnS quantum dots and as low as 0.5 ng/mL for total PSA using an AuNSh-labeled test strip (Srinivasan, Nanus, Erickson, & Mehta, 2021).

These tests demonstrate many of the qualities which would make them fit for a limited purpose like initial screening to exclude one sinister cause of lower urinary tract dysfunction. The costs of such tests are estimated to be circa ~ USD$1 as of the time of writing and could form a useful part of the teleurologists toolkit. While an entirely quantitative high sensitivity test for point-of-need testing is being developed, the initial barrier to the adoption of these LFTs is completing preparatory work for submission of these devices and approval by regulatory bodies such as the FDA and European Medicines Agency (EMA).

Testosterone

Third-party private companies also offer kits including analysis of free testosterone and dehydroepiandrosterone from saliva samples—such as EverlyWell.com, in their "Men's Health Test," which also includes analysis of cortisol and estradiol levels. However, these are not point-of-need tests and require the kit to be sent back to a centralized lab, where EverlyWell.com report that results will be made available "within days" of returning your kit to them (https://www.everlywell.com/products/mens-health-test).

Other providers in this space include Cerascreen (results take 3–5 days, Testosterone Test ~ USD $59), Everywell for $49 LetsGetChecked, myLAB Box (multiple tests including T for $259, results within five days), Verisana ($49 for T test alone), and ZRT Labs. (Pricing as of June 2022).

Similarly, lateral flow immunoassays can be created to test testosterone levels. Similar limitations exist, in that these tests can either be binary—for example, is total testosterone above 300 ng/dL? Or is testosterone greater than 50 ng/dL? Or they can be semiquantitative, in that they can be used in parallel or serial to determine levels <50 ng/dL, between 50 ng/dL and 300 ng/dL, or >300 ng/dL for instance (Miocevic et al., 2017).

Creatinine and eGFR estimation

POC creatinine devices allow rapid measurement of creatinine levels and calculation of estimated glomerular filtration rate (eGFR). This can show whether the kidneys are working properly. This is of particular importance in not just routine monitoring of renal function but also in circumstances where patients may be referred for imaging that also includes contrast, or to assess for an acute or chronic kidney injury in patients with LUTS.

Approved devices include the i-STAT Alinity from Abbott, which is a handheld device that can measure multiple parameters from 65 mL of blood and provide a measurement within 2 min and the Nova Biomedical Stat Sensor, another handheld device that measures creatinine from 1.2 mL of sample within 30 seconds. However, true point-of-need testing devices are not approved or available at the time of writing.

Any blood test

According to the FDA 510k database of over-the-counter (OTC) tests, there are currently no FDA-approved, point-of-need tests for other commonly requested lab values such as hemoglobin, C-reactive protein, or white blood cell count. In theory, these assays are entirely possible; however, as of yet they have not been developed. There are numerous research papers characterizing lateral flow assays to detect thrombin, troponin I, HBsAg, and human immunodeficiency virus (HIV) (Koczula & Gallotta, 2016; Sajid, Kawde, & Daud, 2015). There are numerous providers who offer mail in kits providing lab results in a number of days which have already been discussed earlier in this chapter.

STI checks

Similar to the services described above, there are several mail-in services, who test for sexually transmitted infections such as chlamydia, gonorrhea, HIV, and herpes. These include Everlywell, LetsGetChecked, and QuestDirect.

Urine

Dipstick urinalysis/apps

In the 1950s, single glucose urinalysis was made possible using a paper-based dipstick through enzymatic oxidation of chromogen, followed by commercial introduction in the 1960s. Multiple manufacturers offer urinalysis kits for sale, including over the counter (OTC) in many pharmacies at prices circa $15 USD for 100 strips, albeit sometimes with less information than is typically available from the test strips commonly used in hospital settings. The main reason for this appears to be unit costs balanced with the tests that the majority of consumers are using the strip for.

There are now also a number of FDA-approved urinalysis kits that pair with a mobile app for interpretation and record keeping, such as Healthy.io who call their urinalysis kit application "Dip.io." It was reported to be the first approval of such a test that uses optical equipment designed by a third party (aka your smartphone manufacturer). It examines 10 parameters and can be used for a multitude of purposes from detecting urinary tract infections, chronic kidney disease, and prenatal checks. The parameters tested are: leukocytes (negative or 15/70/125/500 leukocytes/μL), nitrates (negative or positive), glucose (negative or 100/250/500/1000 mg/dL), ketones (negative or 5/15/40/80 mg/dL), protein (negative or 15/30/100/300 mg/dL), blood (negative or 10/25/80/200 erythrocytes/μL), pH (5.0, 5.5, 6.0, 6.5, 7.0, 7.5, 8.0, 8.5, or 9.0), urobilinogen (negative or 1/2/4/8 mg/dL), bilirubin (negative or 1/2/4 mg/dL), and specific gravity (1.000, 1.005, 1.010, 1.015, 1.020,

1.025, or 1.030). The company seems to have made a strategic change, and in early July 2022 received FDA approval for Minuteful Kidney, which is their focused urine dipstick to assess urine albumin to creatinine ratio, and they are awaiting FDA approval of a combined mobile health app and dipstick test focused on diagnosing and monitoring urinary tract infections, and another kit specifically focused on pre-natal care. The company also has reported ambitions to utilize smartphones more fully and incorporate spectroscopy including analysis of infrared and ultraviolet light, which could extend utility to infection control.

There are other providers that couple a urine dipstick with a smartphone app, who are not focused on any one particular medical condition, but may be useful for kidney stone patients owing to the composition of their dipstick test. For example, *Vivoo* (https://vivoo.io/) market their at-home urinalysis strip and mobile app to provide personalized nutrition and lifestyle advice. It should be noted that this is not an FDA or EMA-approved test. It does provide results for the presence of calcium, magnesium, pH, specific gravity (which it labels as hydration) as well as vitamin C, salinity, "oxidative stress," ketones, and protein. The product is sold as a subscription service. Again, it is important to note that this is not an approved test, and its mention here is not an endorsement, but rather as evidence of feasibility, and that measures of interest to urologists, and relevant to the care of urological pa-tients, can be detected and quantified to some degree, with noninvasive tests that are suitable for mobile health applications, and for use by patients in their own home.

The use of urine as a noninvasive test medium to monitor health and detect dis-ease is primed for further development, and is an area where urologists are well placed to lead, and indeed incorporate its use into daily practice. Urine is a relevant analyte not just for urological conditions, benign or malignant, but for many others, as urine contains a wide range of biomarkers already in everyday use. A group in Korea has recently described their efforts to further develop a "lab in a cup," incor-porating the conventional paper-based urine dipstick, already placed in a disposable cup, which is coupled with a smartphone application that automates the analysis pro-cedure. Still in the development stage, the investigators successfully applied their design and application to the detection of glucose, pH, protein, and red blood cells (Rahman, Uddin, Hong, Bhuiyan, & Shim, 2022).

Flow rates/basic urodynamics

The current standard practice of uroflowmetry in urology is equipment, clinic staff, and clinic space-intensive. It requires specialized hardware, consumes time of healthcare workers in preparing the equipment, the space and cleaning each of these afterward, as well as requiring a dedicated space for the procedure in the clinic. A number of researchers have proposed solutions, and MenHealth have received FDA clearance for their MyUroFlow application to address all of the above issues. The application uses the array microphones on the patient's smartphone, android or iOS. To perform a uroflow, the user opens the application on their phone while next to the toilet, presses start and allows it to calibrate for background ambient noise, then urinates as they normally would. The application provides a peak flow rate, voiding volume, and voiding time, and automatically compiles a voiding diary. The application provides a cloud-based dashboard and allows patients to share their results with their urologist. MenHealth (https://myuroflow.com) currently price the application at $15 per month for patients who want to track their flow rates themselves, and provide health practitioners the ability to provide accounts to their patients with provider plans, with per patient prices of $2.50–$5 per month, depending on the number of patients the provider aims to provide the service to.

Soundable Health have developed and released the *proudP* app for Apple iPhones, but it is not currently approved by regulators in the European Union (EU) or United States of America (https://www.soundable.health). The application employs a similar approach and provides max flow rates and voided volumes to patients and providers via an online dashboard. There are also other applications that integrate with hardware devices which must be provided to or purchased by patients, such as iCarePath, which is discussed in more detail in the next chapter.

Diagnostic imaging
Ultrasound and PVR
A number of well-known healthcare device manufacturers have miniature probes, which can be linked to a smartphone or tablet device to provide a portable ultrasound solution. In 2011, Mobisante was the first smartphone-powered ultrasound device to receive FDA approval for its MobiUS SP1 Ultrasound system. Clarius have a range of wireless miniature scanners for use by healthcare professionals (HCPs), which would be of utility to urologists who perform ultrasound as part of their practice. GE Healthcare recently added the Vscan Air to their product catalog. The Vscan Air also connects wirelessly to your smartphone or tablet and received FDA clearance in November 2020. All of these devices require an in-person visit and operation by a trained professional. They do provide the proof of concept that the hardware required to perform ultrasound can be miniaturized and connected to almost ubiquitous communication devices like smartphones and tablets, and pave a path toward low-cost devices, which could be used by patients to perform basic assessments, such as measurement of postvoid residual volume, or even testicular ultrasound and basic kidney imaging.

Advanced imaging
Most advanced imaging is available at standalone imaging centers, which in parts of the United States of America and EU have become not infrequent additions to suburban shopping malls and health centers. They provide an option for medical practitioners to refer patients to often less crowded and more conveniently located

diagnostic services, and can be easily integrated into a telehealth practice workflow. Of particular interest to some is the possibility to have your preferred imaging protocol used by the imaging center, so that if you aim to have the images read by a radiologist separate from that imaging center, or compared with prior imaging, that identical acquisition protocols can be used and compared.

Conclusions

Telemedicine offers much promise, but as with most things, it is how it is executed that will ultimately matter. This platform and infrastructure afford us a relatively rare opportunity to redesign the systems that so often frustrate us, and so often frustrate patients. I do not know of an urologist or any physician who has not been frustrated by the steps, and hoops and ladders, and often seemingly unnecessary measures required to be taken, in order to complete, what at the surface, appear to be relatively simple tasks. For many, it is a simple process to help a patient from the waiting room to have their weight, height, and vitals measured, get a specimen container, and provide them the time and facilities to provide a urine specimen, have a urinalysis completed, flow rate estimation, and postvoid residual scan performed. But more often, this process can involve an administrative staff member to check the patient in, verify their identification, enter their insurance information if they didn't leave it at home, and complete compliance paperwork to process their health information. Then asking the patient to wait for a HCP to help perform measurements, vitals, and clinical specimens, getting administrative assistance in printing and labeling specimens making sure not to confuse them with those of another patient, ensuring sufficient space and privacy for the patient to go to the bathroom, and that they actually have a sufficiently full bladder to perform a useful test at that very moment when the precious space and time constrained HCP is available. And all of that is before they ever actually get as far as seeing the doctor they came to see. I think a simple survey of physicians in practice asking: 'have you ever had a patient respond to a name that wasn't theirs?', would provide sufficient evidence to demonstrate how the current system could be refined. If we were to ask clinicians, have you ever seen a patient who had been booked for the wrong investigation or even procedure, the answers would provide sufficient proof that the current systems in use are deficient and unfit for purpose.

That is not to say there is a carte blanche for physicians to institute whatever they want. While there are government regulations currently in place, many of them were not designed for a telehealthcare system. New regulations will be required, some existing regulations will be made redundant, and others will need to be revised. It is imperative though that all stakeholders meaningfully engage with this process. Physicians have traditionally allowed this process to occur in their absence; they must now ensure they are front and center to design the system that best serves all patients. This is an opportunity to design a healthcare system, knowing the strengths, limitations, opportunities, and vulnerabilities of multiple systems, which operated in a physical space over centuries. We can now build one in a metaphysical space, with all the knowledge gained from the real world, and are the best placed group to help do this.

The Health Insurance Portability and Accountability Act (HIPAA) is the perfect example of a law requiring thorough revision in an age of telemedicine. HIPAA is widely known as the piece of legislation in the United States of America that protects patient's privacy rights, as it applies to how healthcare providers, health insurers, and clearinghouses handle some patient data. What is critical to clarify though is that HIPAA only applies to those specific entities that also receive federal funds—for example, by processing payments for patients using Medicare and Medicaid. It does not apply to entirely private practices. HIPAA also does not apply to thousands of apps, digital devices, fitness devices, or wellness apps, which record our behavior, track our activity, or measure our vital signs and biometric data. While HIPAA does not allow health plans or healthcare providers to sell personal, identifiable health data, it does not regulate what other entities do with these data. Mobile devices, wearable health trackers, and connected home devices are now as commonplace in the lives of Americans as a toaster, and the exploitation of such data has been well documented.

Bibliography

Arpaia, P., Cimmino, P., De Matteis, E., Montenero, G., & Manna, G. C. (2012). Integrated telemedicine systems: Patient monitoring, in-time prognostics, and diagnostics at domicile. In *The design and manufacture of medical devices* (pp. 273–328). Elsevier.

Bock, S., An, J., Kim, H. M., Kim, J., Jung, H. S., Pham, X. H., ... Jun, B. H. (2020). A lateral flow immunoassay for prostate-specific antigen detection using silica-coated CdSe @ ZnS quantum dots. *Bulletin of the Korean Chemical Society, 41*(10), 989–993. https://doi.org/10.1002/bkcs.12099

Charlton, G. (2020). *What are the peak times for online shopping?*. Retrieved from https://www.thedrum.com/opinion/2020/02/27/what-are-the-peak-times-online-shopping.

Hutchison, R. (1998). Favourite prayers: The physician's prayer. *BMJ: British Medical Journal, 317*, 1687. https://doi.org/10.1136/bmj.317.7174.1687a. https://www.bmj.com/content/317/7174/1687.2

Johnson, E. K., Estrada, C. R., Johnson, K. L., Nguyen, H. T., Rosoklija, I., & Nelson, C. P. (2014). Evaluation of a mobile voiding diary for pediatric patients with voiding dysfunction: A prospective comparative study. *The Journal of Urology, 192*(3), 908–913. https://doi.org/10.1016/j.juro.2014.03.099

Koczula, K. M., & Gallotta, A. (2016). Lateral flow assays. *Essays in Biochemistry, 60*(1), 111–120. https://doi.org/10.1042/EBC20150012

Leone, M. J., Fernandez Slezak, D., Golombek, D., & Sigman, M. (2017). Time to decide: Diurnal variations on the speed and quality of human decisions. *Cognition, 158*, 44–55. https://doi.org/10.1016/j.cognition.2016.10.007

Linhares, B. L., Miranda, E. P., Cintra, A. R., Reges, R., & Torres, L. O. (2021). Use, misuse and abuse of testosterone and other androgens. *Sexual Medicine Reviews*. https://doi.org/10.1016/j.sxmr.2021.10.002

Miano, R., Mele, G. O., Germani, S., Bove, P., Sansalone, S., Pugliese, P. F., & Micali, F. (2005). Evaluation of a new, rapid, qualitative, one-step PSA test for prostate cancer screening: The PSA RapidScreen test. *Prostate Cancer and Prostatic Diseases, 8*(3), 219–223. https://doi.org/10.1038/sj.pcan.4500802

Miocevic, O., Cole, C. R., Laughlin, M. J., Buck, R. L., Slowey, P. D., & Shirtcliff, E. A. (2017). Quantitative lateral flow assays for salivary biomarker assessment: A review. *Frontiers in Public Health, 5*, 133. https://doi.org/10.3389/fpubh.2017.00133

Rahman, M. M., Uddin, M. J., Hong, J. H., Bhuiyan, N. H., & Shim, J. S. (2022). Lab-in-a-Cup (LiC): An autonomous fluidic device for daily urinalysis using smartphone. *Sensors and Actuators B: Chemical, 355*. https://doi.org/10.1016/j.snb.2021.131336

Sajid, M., Kawde, A.-N., & Daud, M. (2015). Designs, formats and applications of lateral flow assay: A literature review. *Journal of Saudi Chemical Society, 19*(6), 689–705. https://doi.org/10.1016/j.jscs.2014.09.001

Srinivasan, B., Nanus, D. M., Erickson, D., & Mehta, S. (2021). Highly portable quantitative screening test for prostate-specific antigen at point of care. *Current Research in Biotechnology, 3*, 288–299. https://doi.org/10.1016/j.crbiot.2021.11.003

Willis, B. H., Beebee, H., & Lasserson, D. S. (2013). Philosophy of science and the diagnostic process. *Family Practice, 30*(5), 501–505. https://doi.org/10.1093/fampra/cmt031

Remote patient monitoring in urology

Introduction

Digital sensors and devices are in widespread use to monitor many physiologic functions. They provide indicators and parameters for early warning scores for patients in acute health systems, whether as telemetry, continuous pulse and oximetry, urine output, and other sensor systems. In many parts or the world, such monitoring systems are in widespread use, but their use could be expanded right now, to include other settings; where the patient is in a step-down unit, or ambulatory care facility, or even at home. In a similar fashion to their use in hospitals, such digital sensors can be used to provide an objective measure of a subject's status and also provide indicators of whether or not a patient is deteriorating or improving. These could be used, and would be of utility to monitor patients with chronic conditions or to monitor patients postoperatively after discharge from a health facility; enabling early intervention, and perhaps improving patient outcomes and reducing hospital readmissions.

There are opportunities to use telehealth tools to engage patients with their health and the health system after they leave the hospital, and even to prevent admission to hospital. At the University Of Michigan Department Of Urology, an automated chat bot was used to provide postoperative instructions to patients after ureteroscopy (Modi, Portney, Hollenbeck, & Ellimoottil, 2018). While such work is an area of ongoing research, healthcare providers must be careful that they don't neglect to interact with their patients, and defer important postoperative care (and indeed preoperative care and consenting), to automated digital tools. Such misuse of technology may significantly impact on patient outcomes and act to undermine the physician—patient relationship; replacing it with something more akin to a customer—provider relationship. Medical ethicists have long decried the impact of economic pushes and pulls in medical practice and the challenges they provide to the physician—patient relationship (Veatch, 1997) (Emanuel, 1992). Using telemedicine to engage patients after they leave the hospital or doctor's office is an area of ongoing research, and has significant potential to improve the value of healthcare by providing information and reassurance to patients. This chapter will focus more on systems, strategies, and devices that decrease the distance and barriers, and enable ongoing engagement with their physician.

Challenges in remote patient monitoring (RPM) include making patients comfortable with the technology and the constant monitoring. A large component of this is patient education, which in many settings, is largely performed by those coordinating care, whether physicians, nurses, or allied health professionals. This window for patient education, often is best suited to take place when the patient is admitted to a healthcare facility, and they can become familiar with the device and troubleshoot any issues that may arise. This is preferable to the scenario, where patient discharge is imminent, and the device is handed over to the patient, with minimal time for them to interact and become comfortable with it. With time though, it should be the case that minimal to no further patient education is required, and that such monitoring systems are either completely autonomous or are innately intuitive, and require minimal to no conscious user input, so that anybody can benefit from their use.

Other challenges to RPM range from upfront costs and capital expenditure for suitable devices, licenses, and infrastructure to reimbursement for telemonitoring. There is due concern that the digital divide will become more apparent and that while telemonitoring may help reduce some disparities (for example, rural vs. urban dwellers), other disparities may be magnified. The field is very much in its infancy, and for more complex conditions, the field is still identifying optimal patient groups that would benefit. However, for routine care and preventing readmissions, the case can be made that all that is missing is the will to implement telemonitoring.

Benefits of remote monitoring
Prevent readmissions

Almost 20 years ago, the Veterans Health Administration, a nationalized healthcare service in the United States, introduced a national home telehealth program which is known as "Care Coordination/Home Telehealth" (CCHT). The Veterans Heath Association is the largest integrated healthcare system in the United States of America and provides care to over nine million military veterans at over 1200 healthcare facilities.

The CCHT coordinates the management of chronic conditions and was launched with the objective of reducing and preventing unnecessary hospital admissions. The service is a small part of the overall Veteran Health Administration; the CCHT was initially staffed by over 5000 trained staff, a small fraction of the over 350,000 employed by the Veteran Health Affairs. The CCHT systematizes the implementation of health informatics, home telehealth, and disease management technologies. In a study published on data obtained from 17,025 patients enrolled in CCHT, there was a 25% reduction in number of bed days of care, 19% reduction in hospital admissions, and a mean satisfaction score rating of 86% (Darkins et al., 2008). The impact of this work is all the more meaningful to patients, especially those who wish to remain in their own home and live independently. During this study which was conducted between July 2003 and December 2007, the cost of this service was $1600 per annum. This pales in comparison with the figure reported by the United States Government Accountability Office in a 2020 report on Veterans Affairs (VA) Health Care, which reported the average cost per day for veteran's care as $268 in a community nursing home, and $1074 per day in a VA community living center. This is all the more considerable, when VA data show that the number of veterans receiving long-term care in VA funded programs was 530,327 in 2018, a sizable portion of the over nine million veterans the Veteran Health Administration provides care to. Over 5% of veterans discharged from hospital are discharged to a long-term care facility (Burke, Canamucio, Glorioso, Baron, & Ryskina, 2019). This is a sizable burden, and CCHT and its remote monitoring program were able to reduce the number of hospital days by ∼25% in this population with high healthcare utility, for a cost between 1/60th and 1/240th of long term care (Table 8.1).

CCHT's program demonstrated very tangible benefits, and was received positively by the majority of the patients to whom it was offered. Only 10% of over 17,000 patients it was offered to, declined to take part in the program. The high patient satisfaction of the CCHT program in the United States is consistent with other programs elsewhere around the world, from Europe to Asia (Lu, Chi, & Chen, 2014; Zanaboni, Knarvik, & Wootton, 2014).

Improve patient care

An often-overlooked performance indicator is patient access. Patients who are otherwise unable to access, or have limited access to care, are by virtue of not having access, excluded from the metric. When considering anecdotes, discussions and studies on remote patient monitoring, keep in mind that much of the existing

Table 8.1 Cost of a remote monitoring program offered by the United States Veteran Health Service compared with costs for their home-based primary care services, average costs of community nursing home and average costs of a Veteran Affairs Community Living Center care.

	Cost per day	Cost per month	Cost per year
VA CCHT	$ 4.38	$ 133.33	$ 1600.00
VHA home-based primary care services	$ 35.95	$ 1093.42	$ 13,121.00
Community nursing home	$ 269.00	$ 8182.08	$ 98,185.00
VA community living center	$ 1074	$ 32,667.50	$ 392,010

CCHT, *care coordination/home telehealth;* VA, *veteran affairs;* VHA, *veteran health affairs.*
Sources *https://www.gao.gov/assets/gao-20-284.pdf and (Darkins, A., Ryan, P., Kobb, R., Foster, L., Edmonson, E., Wakefield, B., & Lancaster, A. E. (2008). Care coordination/home telehealth: The systematic implementation of health informatics, home telehealth, and disease management to support the care of veteran patients with chronic conditions.* Telemedicine Journal and e-Health, 14(10), 1118 −1126. 10.1089/tmj.2008.0021).

experience and data, only accounts for those who have already had access, and may not be representative of all patients.

Telemonitoring and stable disease clinics

Boyd Viers et al. conducted a randomized and controlled trial assessing telehealth clinics compared with in-person clinics in patients who had undergone radical prostatectomy. In total, 70 patients were randomized and 55 completed their visit. Nonattendance was 25% (9/36) for the in-person visit, and 18% (6/34) for the telehealth clinic (Viers et al., 2015).

In this study, they considered efficiency as total time spent on patient care, and found no difference between either modality (mean 17.9 vs. 17.8 min, 95% CI 5.9 to 5.6; $P = .97$). The total clinician–patient contact time (12.1 vs. 11.8 min, 95% CI 4.2 to 3.5; $P = .85$), and patient wait time (18.4 vs 13.0 min, 95% CI 13.7 to 3.0; $P = .20$), were also no different between the study arms.

Furthermore, there was no difference in patient satisfaction in the telehealth group ($n = 21/24$, 88%) compared with the in-person group ($n = 20/22$, 91%; $P = .70$). Uniquely, Viers et al. also recorded clinician satisfaction, with 88% of telehealth and 90% of in-person clinic urologists reporting "very good" or "excellent" ratings. Most (88%) of the telehealth patients (21/24), and 73% of patients in the in-person group (16/22), strongly agreed (Likert scale 1–7), that they could be seen without physical examination for every appointment, addressing a common telehealth concern.

However, as well as power limitations, there was a risk of selection bias, as only 24% (70/295) of screened men were randomized. After prescreening, reasons for noneligibility included 70/155 patients (45%) who declined (reasons unstated), 25 patients (16%) lacking capable technologies, 15 patients (10%) uncomfortable with a telehealth visit, and 15 patients (8%) requesting in-person consultation for medical reasons, limiting its generalizability. Finally, the end totals for the telehealth and in-person groups decreased to 24 and 22, respectively (i.e., nine men were not included); ideally the authors could have adopted an intention-to-treat analysis. In a Scottish study of a nurse-led prostate cancer follow-up clinic delivered by telehealth, Robertson et al. [2013], surveys were sent to 302 men. Eligibility criteria included patients if they had prostate-specific antigen (PSA)-stable disease, were a minimum of 2 years postradiotherapy, and had been seen already in an in-person clinic for $\geq$6 months. Patients were followed-up every 6-months for 3 years, then annually for 5 years, and then reviewed at 10 years if there were no consecutive PSA rises. The study protocol included that the clinical nurse specialist met weekly with an oncologist to discuss patients with PSA rises. As part of this study, patients visited their general practitioner (GP) for laboratory investigations every 6 months, and were informed of results by letter from the reviewing clinical nurse specialists (along with their GP). In this study, Robertson et al. reported that 50 in-person appointments were saved per month following the introduction of this telehealth delivered follow up program. Surveys were performed to assess patient satisfaction with this service, and a total of 191 surveys (63.2%) were returned. These showed that 98.4%

of men were happy with the new telehealth service, and 98.8% felt "well supported" by it. This study does have it's limitations though, and the publication does not provide patient demographics, nor does it provide data sufficient to explain how 50 in-person specialist appointments were saved per month.

Wearables and devices

Wearable devices refer to small electronic devices that are worn on bodies and can often take the form of watches, rings, glasses or are integrated into an item of clothing. They are portable and convenient, and sometimes include computing power on-board the device itself, but do not necessarily do so. Wearables in medicine are not a modern phenomenon, as the first wearable hearing aids date back to 1800.

Current technology is primed to enable greater innovation and utilization of these devices and technologies in urology, as there is widespread availability of sensors including: accelerometers, altimeters, digital cameras with charge coupled devices (CCD), electrical capacitors, microphones, infra-red pulse oximeters and photoplethysmography, Bluetooth proximity sensors, pressure sensors, and thermometers integrated into digital devices from cell phones, smartwatches, smart jewelry, and sensors embedded in clothing (Sivani & Mishra, 2022).

Remote monitoring: uroflow and voiding diaries

CarePath have developed a device which can be used by both men and women to record urine output and record uroflow rates. The device communicates with a smart phone and provides the sensor technology required to record void-related data—namely uroflow and voided volume. Data are connected to a cloud server where flow rate and volume calculations are performed and stored in a HIPAA-compliant fashion, as per the device manufacturer. CarePath recommend that the patient use the device every time that they void urine, and that males and females be seated to use the device. CarePath state that information gathered on the first day of use is discarded as the patient becomes familiar with the device.

The system comes with a number of components and maybe cumbersome and "involved" for many patients. The device itself needs some basic assembly before use and has reusable and disposable components. The CarePath device handle is reusable and contains a rechargeable battery. This needs to be attached to a disposable component, which receives the urine flow. There is also a base station that also acts as a charging station for the handheld device and a mobile app to which the device must be paired in order to communicate to the cloud servers that process the data and maintain a voiding diary.

The device and its use does require some setup and manual dexterity to assemble the device before each use, as well as holding the device handle and correctly orienting it as the patient sits for each urine void, and this may be problematic for some (Fig. 8.1).

MyUroFlow from MenHealth is another mobile application offering to help monitor urine flow rates and voided volume. MenHealth offers a mobile app and

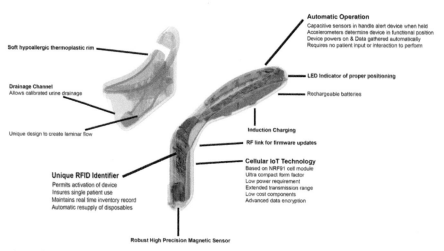

FIGURE 8.1

Carepath's remote patient monitoring device allowing for estimation of flow rate and helping to log voided urine volumes.

Image from https://i-ourology.com/rpm-urology/

web portal. The solution offered utilizes the microphone on the user's smartphone and analyzes the sound of urine flow as it hits the water in the toilet, thus enabling measurement of urinary flow rate, and estimation of voided volume.

MyUroflow is a Food and Drug Administration—cleared application and was tested in men older than 18 years. A study of 62 patients comparing the MyUroFlow app used by patients at home to standard Prometheus Office Uroflowmetry noted that 4 participants did not operate the MyUroFlow app properly, similar to four who could not properly perform the standard in office uroflowmetry. The study also demonstrated that there was no statistically significant difference between the two modalities (Tavrovsky & Schultz, 2021) (Fig. 8.2).

Remote patient monitoring postoperatively

Postoperative RPM has emerged as a promising technology to improve the quality and safety of surgical care. By providing real-time data on patient's vital signs and clinical status, RPM can help surgeons and other clinicians to optimize postoperative management, and identify early signs of complications. A number of studies have demonstrated the feasibility and potential benefits of RPM in various surgical specialties, including urology.

In a study of postoperative RPM in urology, Kavoussi et al. found that RPM was associated with a significant reduction in length of stay and 30-day readmission rates. The authors also found that RPM was associated with improved surgical

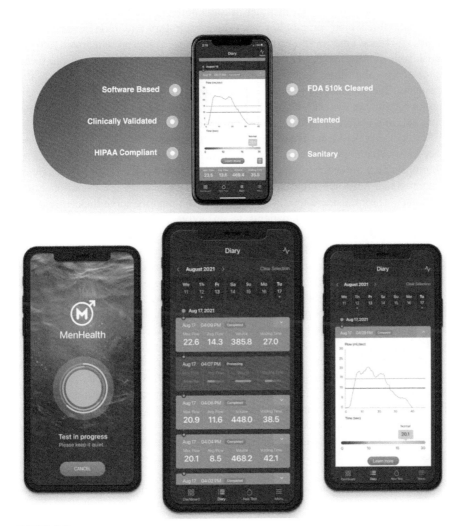

FIGURE 8.2

Overview of the application MyUroFlow which uses the array microphones on contemporary smartphones to estimate voided urine volume.

Image source = https://myuroflow.com

outcomes, as measured by the Clavien–Dindo classification system. These findings suggest that RPM may be a valuable tool for improving the quality of surgical care in urology.

Other digital health and device manufacturers are also helping to not only provide the tools for RPM, but also collaborating to conduct clinical trials into their utility. One such collaboration is that between Somahealth, Mount Sinai Hospitals in

New York and the Karolinska Instituet in Stockholm. The RPM solution incorporates a wearable which can monitor heart rate, respiratory rate, blood oxygen saturations, and blood glucose among other measurements, which are integrated into the Somahealth monitoring center. The monitoring center is a cloud-based platform, augmented by algorithms which analyze patient data and also provide alerts to the care team. The collaboration involving Urology departments in Mount Sinai and Karolinska aims to evaluate if readmissions can be reduced, and patient outcomes improved, in a cohort of patients undergoing radical cystectomy.

Postoperative RPM has also been examined following a wide variety of other procedures, which integrate measurements which are of relevance to patients undergoing urological procedures. The ŒDIPE trial examined the safety and efficacy of an abbreviated hospitalization after implantation or replacement of dual-chamber pacemakers (PMs), using a telecardiology-based ambulatory surveillance program. This trial randomly assigned patients to an active group who were discharged 24 hours after their first PM implant, or 4–6 hours after replacement, and followed for 4 weeks with remote telemonitoring in their home, or patients were randomly assigned to the control group followed for 4 weeks as per routine care. The primary objective of the ŒDIPE trial was to confirm that the proportion of patients who experienced one or more major adverse events (MAE) was not higher in the active (remote telemonited) group than in the control (routine care) group. This study included 379 patients who had a dual chamber pacemaker inserted. MAE rate was similar between study groups, and at least one treatment-related MAE was observed in 9.2% of patients ($n = 17$) assigned to the active group, versus 13.3% of patients ($n = 26$) in the control group ($P = 0.21$).   Even though this is normally a procedure associated with a single night in hospital, the mean hospitalization duration was 34% shorter in the active arm than in the control group ($P < 0.001$). This study of patients undergoing cardiac pacemaker placement demonstrated that remote monitoring by telehealth allowed for the early detection of adverse events, and provides further evidence as to the feasibility and utility of remote patient monitoring (Halimi et al., 2008).

A Canadian study conducted by Kuper and Van Koughnett in 46 colorectal surgery patients, examined the feasibility of home monitoring using a daily automated survey and wound photo upload delivered by a mobile health app. Patients undergoing colorectal surgery are typically older, and so this is of particular relevance to a large swath of the urology patient population, and maybe helpful to answer the question posed by many, as to whether such systems would be acceptable to an older patient population. The study measured patient compliance, patient satisfaction with the remote monitoring program, and the association between generated alerts and readmission rate. Patient compliance was defined as the frequency of patients completing study-related tasks on each postdischarge day among those patients still being followed in the study. Feasibility was predefined as acceptable, if 80% of patients completed a daily survey or wound photo upload 80% of the time. In addition to these criteria, at least 80% of readmissions needed to be preceded by an alert or wound photo on the day of, or the day prior to readmission, for the study intervention to be deemed feasible. While this appears to be an arbitrary definition, it isn't expected that this definition would satisfy most surgeon's definition of adequate postoperative review. In this study of colorectal patients from Western Canada, 37.0% of patients answered the survey at least 80% of the time, in the first 2 weeks following discharge. The authors assign this to "poor compliance" with answering the daily survey, and also noted that compliance diminished over the two-week period, where compliance reduced by 5.9% every 7 days, and where only 17.4% of the patients $n = 8/46$) responded to the survey every day. A similar number did not respond to the survey at all, over the same period. This is particularly interesting as over 86% were smartphone or tablet owners and over 84% were computer or laptop owners, and over 71% of participants reported daily use of a smartphone or tablet. It is as equally surprising given the low compliance that patient satisfaction was high; 80.5% of patients reported that they felt safer going home knowing that they were monitored, and 76.2% of patients reported that they would use the current app for postoperative monitoring again. It seems this study had significant limitations, and that perhaps there was suboptimal patient understanding of the nature of the remote monitoring, but it does provide some interesting insights into what is acceptable to patients, and what is practical if the aim is to provide meaningful patient care remotely.

While this study does act as somewhat of a cautionary tale, it does provide many meaningful and useful findings. Another of which is that the investigators had initially planned to track postoperative recovery of preoperative activity levels, using activity trackers; however, the activity trackers did not consistently sync with the mobile health app being utilized for this study, and the authors report measurements were found to be inaccurate (Kuper, 2020). This yet again highlights that as with all devices, technically advanced or otherwise, that usability, reliability, and security remain as fundamental basic functions, which otherwise competent investigators can overlook. Such systems will require extensive testing and validation before being implemented, and bootstrapped systems can act to impede progress rather than offer meaningful solutions which can be broadly adopted. I applaud the investigators for their efforts to advance the field and their honesty in reporting this important work.

There are a number of devices which can be integrated for specific purposes which may be of utility for postoperative RPM. The Ostom-i is a novel device that helps patients with colostomies monitor their stoma output (see Fig. 9.1). The principles underlying the sensor do not preclude it from urological applications, such as measuring urine output. The creators of the device claim it is the world's first connected device for stoma care. The device uses a sensor to measure the weight of the stoma output, and then sends this information to a smartphone app. The app then uses an algorithm to calculate the total volume of output and sends this information to the patient. The device has been shown to be accurate within ±5% of the total volume of output. The device is currently in clinical trials and has been shown to be well tolerated by patients. A study of the usability of the device in a cohort of 9 patients was performed by Kontovounisios et al. (2018). This study was conducted

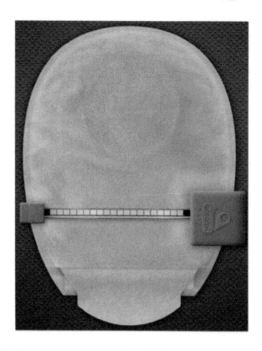

FIGURE 8.3

Ostom-i sensor attached to a stoma bag (Kontovounisios et al., 2018). The device is CE-marked and FDA approved as a medical device. It is composed of a flexible sensor which detects stoma bag filling and communicates that information to a paired smart phone application.

while patients were in-patients, and while there were issues with network connectivity when patients changed ward in the hospital, they did describe that patients were able to pair the device and remove and reattach the device without difficulty. While conscious not to present an overly optimistic interpretation of these results, this does demonstrate that functional and useful connected devices exist, which patients in a similar demographic to urology patients are able to use and which would enable remote monitoring of patients who may be recovering from what are considered to be complex procedures(Fig. 8.3).

Bibliography

Burke, R. E., Canamucio, A., Glorioso, T. J., Baron, A. E., & Ryskina, K. L. (2019). Transitional care outcomes in veterans receiving post-acute care in a skilled nursing facility. *Journal of the American Geriatrics Society, 67*(9), 1820–1826. https://doi.org/10.1111/jgs.15971

Darkins, A., Ryan, P., Kobb, R., Foster, L., Edmonson, E., Wakefield, B., & Lancaster, A. E. (2008). Care coordination/home telehealth: The systematic implementation of health informatics, home telehealth, and disease management to support the care of veteran patients with chronic conditions. *Telemedicine Journal and e-Health, 14*(10), 1118—1126. https://doi.org/10.1089/tmj.2008.0021

Emanuel, E. J. (1992). Four models of the physician-patient relationship. *JAMA: The Journal of the American Medical Association, 267*(16), 2221—2226. https://doi.org/10.1001/jama.1992.03480160079038

Halimi, F., Clementy, J., Attuel, P., Dessenne, X., Amara, W., & Investigators, O.t. (2008). Optimized post-operative surveillance of permanent pacemakers by home monitoring: The OEDIPE trial. *Europace, 10*(12), 1392—1399. https://doi.org/10.1093/europace/eun250

Kontovounisios, C., Smith, J., Dawson, P., Warren, O., Mills, S., Von Roon, A., ... Tekkis, P. (2018). The ostom-i alert sensor: A new device to measure stoma output. *Techniques in Coloproctology, 22*(9), 697—701. https://doi.org/10.1007/s10151-018-1846-6

Kuper, T. (2020). *Feasibility of post-operative mobile health monitoring among colorectal surgery patients*. Electronic Thesis and Dissertation Repository (p. 6928). Retrieved from https://ir.lib.uwo.ca/etd/6928.

Lu, J. F., Chi, M. J., & Chen, C. M. (2014). Advocacy of home telehealth care among consumers with chronic conditions. *Journal of Clinical Nursing, 23*(5—6), 811—819. https://doi.org/10.1111/jocn.12156

Modi, P. K., Portney, D., Hollenbeck, B. K., & Ellimoottil, C. (2018). Engaging telehealth to drive value-based urology. *Current Opinion in Urology, 28*(4), 342—347. https://doi.org/10.1097/MOU.0000000000000508

Robertson, A. F., Windsor, P. M., & Smith, A. (2013). *International Journal of Urological Nursing, 7*(2), 92—97. https://doi.org/10.1111/j.1749-771X.2012.01161.x

Sivani, T., & Mishra, S. (2022). Wearable devices: Evolution and usage in remote patient monitoring system. In S. Mishra, A. González-Briones, A. K. Bhoi, P. K. Mallick, & J. M. Corchado (Eds.), *Connected e-health: Integrated IoT and cloud computing* (pp. 311—332). Cham: Springer International Publishing.

Tavrovsky, M., & Schultz, R. E. (2021). Mp02-10 menhealth Uroflowmetry app is equivalent to standard office Uroflowmetry. *Journal of Urology, 206*(Suppl. 3). https://doi.org/10.1097/ju.0000000000001963.10

Veatch, R. M. (1997). *Medical ethics*. Jones and Bartlett Publishers.

Viers, B. R., Lightner, D. J., Rivera, M. E., Tollefson, M. K., Boorjian, S. A., Karnes, R. J., ... Gettman, M. T. (2015). Efficiency, satisfaction, and costs for remote video visits following radical prostatectomy: A randomized controlled trial. *European Urology, 68*(4), 729—735. https://doi.org/10.1016/j.eururo.2015.04.002

Zanaboni, P., Knarvik, U., & Wootton, R. (2014). Adoption of routine telemedicine in Norway: The current picture. *Global Health Action, 7*(1), 22801. https://doi.org/10.3402/gha.v7.22801

Digital therapeutics

Introduction

Remote therapy and digital therapeutics encompass a number of therapeutic modalities, from e-prescribing, remote surgery, eHealth, and virtual care to digital devices as therapies. Digital therapeutics are well suited for the "one-to-many" model of care, where the reach of physicians to treat patients can overcome time, place, and personnel constraints that can limit healthcare access and delivery. Such therapies, whether digitally enabled, digitally enhanced or otherwise, must be as all approved therapies now are: evidence-based, rigorously evaluated with proven safety and efficacy, and appropriately regulated. This section will focus mainly on digital therapeutics which can be delivered remote from the "normal" or usual site of care provision. Remote surgery will be discussed in more detail in the next chapter.

A good framework for considering digital therapeutics as a distinct class is as delivering medical interventions directly to patients to treat, manage, or even prevent disease or dysfunction. There are 10 core principles or criteria that the Digital Therapeutic Alliance list, which must be adhered to in order for a product to be considered a digital therapeutic (Table 9.1).

Many digital therapeutics are regulated as "software as a medical device." Despite the multiple names and forms of such therapies, global regulators have been scrambling to keep pace with how to classify, regulate, and designate such therapies. While the Food and Drug Administration (FDA) has cleared (note the distinction) or approved digital therapeutic products for over a decade now, the European Medicines Agency (at the time of writing) has not yet designated a regulatory pathway for evaluation and commercialization of digital therapeutics. Despite regulatory uncertainties and no clear indication as to whether insurers or payors will cover or reimburse such therapies, companies focused on digital therapeutics have thrived and seen investor interest surge as the COVID-19 pandemic of 2020 disrupted healthcare delivery.

Digital therapeutics also offer many opportunities not just for patients and physicians, but also for health systems. The lower risk profile of many digital therapeutics, as well as lower development costs and shorter duration from concept to commercialization, requires less capital investment. As regulatory uncertainty around digital therapeutics diminishes, digital therapeutics may help lower the costs of healthcare.

Telehealth in Urology. https://doi.org/10.1016/B978-0-323-87480-9.00002-6

Table 9.1 List of 10 core principles that all products claiming to be a digital therapeutic must adhere to as per the Digital Therapeutic Alliance (DTxAlliance.org) https://dtxalliance.org/wp-content/uploads/2021/01/DTA_DTx-Definition-and-Core-Principles.pdf.

1	Prevent, manage, or treat a medical disorder or disease
2	Produce a medical intervention that is driven by software
3	Incorporate design, manufacture, and quality best practices
4	Engage end users in product development and usability processes
5	Incorporate patient privacy and security protections
6	Apply product deployment, management, and maintenance best practices
7	Publish trial results inclusive of clinically meaningful outcomes in peer-reviewed journals
8	Be reviewed and cleared or certified by regulatory bodies as required to support product claims of risk, efficacy, and intended use
9	Make claims appropriate to clinical evaluation and regulatory status
10	Collect, analyze, and apply real-world evidence and/or product performance data

Regulatory considerations for digital therapeutics

While the development of digital therapeutics for urological conditions is in its infancy, other specialties have seen FDA approvals following submission of trial data demonstrating superiority, using both de novo and 510(k) pathways for medical devices. Others, namely Cognoa, who partnered with EVERSANA, received Breakthrough Designation from the FDA for their digital diagnostic and therapeutic for autism spectrum disorder. To put this in context, Breakthrough Designation is awarded by the FDA to help expedite the development and approval of treatments that treat a serious condition and where preliminary clinical evidence indicates that the treatment may demonstrate substantial improvement over available therapies on a clinically significant endpoint. The FDA clarifies that clinically significant endpoints are those that measure an effect on irreversible morbidity (or mortality), further punctuating the recognition that digital therapeutics can disrupt and offer real benefits over pharmaceutical or other treatments, which have been the mainstay of therapy for a number of conditions for over half a century.

The regulatory framework for the approval of digital therapeutic interventions is not as defined as that for physical devices or pharmaceuticals. In 2017, the FDA introduced a Software Precertification Pilot Program which aimed to help inform the development of a regulatory model to assess such innovations. While the FDA has subsequently released discussion documents and draft guidance is available, it is clear that a comprehensive and well-defined pathway requires a great deal of time and many case examples before more certainty exists for those developing such therapies.

In the United States of America, some digital therapeutics must undergo randomized controlled trials under the premarket approval process to demonstrate acceptable safety and efficacy. Digital therapeutics are inherently different though from pharmaceuticals, the form of which remains stable and composition unchanged over time. Many digital therapeutics that are essentially software as a medical device have the potential and indeed often require frequent updates following FDA review, much as the operating system on servers, computers, and smart devices do. Other digital therapeutics that utilize machine learning or other artificial intelligence (AI) as a component may evolve as they "learn" the optimal features over time.

Digital therapeutics in urology

The current field of digital therapeutics is largely focused on chronic conditions or those that are modifiable by means of behavioral change. The therapy, which was otherwise an in-person service, is provided as a digital product which may be over-the-counter or prescription only. Similar to a prescription medicine, the prescription-only digital therapeutic is prescribed and the patient is ultimately directed to the manufacturer who, by various means, enrolls the patient onto the digital therapeutic. Digital therapies often make use of an access code or other time-constrained access modality to enable the use of a mobile application as prescribed and as per the digital therapeutics approved label. Web dashboards are often available, which allow patients and physicians to monitor progress and compliance. While the field of digital therapeutics is still in its infancy, the number of approved and available therapies currently focused on patients exclusively with urological conditions is limited. Throughout this chapter, an overview is provided of digital therapeutics currently approved or in development in contexts which are relevant to urology. While some may currently be approved for specific conditions, they are of utility to the care of patients with urological complaints, which may benefit the urologist in helping to provide more holistic care and may even provide inspiration for adaption and help improve care of patients with other conditions.

Example use cases of digital therapeutics
Preventative care

Livongo is a digital therapeutic product for diabetes, diabetes prevention, weight management, and hypertension. It is, however, not FDA approved. It is still commercially available though. Livongo is operated by Teladoc Health, a large virtual care company, which says they are "creating a truly unified and personalized consumer experience; developing technologies to connect to patients and extend the reach of care providers; delivering the highest standard of clinical quality at every touchpoint; and enhancing health decisions and outcomes with smart data and actionable insights." They are by their own description a consumer company, and despite their name, are not a health company. The underlying concept though, allows for preventative care which is relevant to those with metabolic syndrome, for example, a condition highly prevalent amongst urology patients—and was present in ∼39% in a study conducted in male urology patients (Bal et al., 2007).

Wellthy CARE Digital Therapeutics Platform also provides an offering for lifestyle modification and enables weight loss in patients with obesity and metabolic syndrome. They offer a yearlong program, which includes a health coach, supports for diet modification, physical activity, and remote patient monitoring of glycemic control and blood pressure. They conducted a single arm study involving 196 participants over a period of 52 weeks (Adhikary et al., 2021). While there was no control arm, those who were in the highest quartile in terms of app engagement lost 3 kg of weight compared to those in the lowest quartile who lost 1.2 kg. While further work is required to fully validate this specific platform, it does offer a positive signal of the potential utility of such interventions in preventative care.

Preoperative assessment

Urologic patients undergoing surgical procedures require careful preoperative evaluation and planning prior to surgery. Failure to assess the preoperative needs of these patients could potentially lead to increased intraoperative and/or postoperative morbidity. The effect may be temporary, such as increased postoperative dementia in geriatric patients taking certain preoperative medications (Jeong et al., 2016), or more insidious, as seen with increased complications in patients with suboptimal nutrition prior to radical cystectomy (Johnson et al., 2016). In addition to increased morbidity, an incomplete preoperative assessment can have financial implications for both the patient and the hospital system. For example, a prospective cross-sectional study from 2011 looked at surgical cancellation rates in 25 hospitals and found that approximately 8% of elective urological surgeries were canceled and rescheduled within 24 h of the scheduled procedure (Schuster et al., 2011). Medical administrative reasons, such as incomplete medical work, have been cited as a major source of many of the cancellations. Such digital tools and therapies can help improve patient compliance with pre-operative care instructions, and with nutritional status, and even help in the completion of the pre-operative assessment itself.

Managing chronic conditions

Another robot doing in the rounds is Catalia Health's Mabu. Mabu, an abbreviated form of the Japanese word "Mabudachi", meaning close friend, uses AI and psychological modeling to encourage and motivate people to take their medications. It isn't just an alarm clock on wheels, but it aims to build relationships with patients and customizes its conversations to keep patients adhering to dosing regimens for longer. It is currently being used in helping patients with congestive heart failure, rheumatoid arthritis, chronic kidney disease as well as being integrated into clinical trials to help record and report patient reported outcomes and improve treatment adherence in ambulatory trials. It can also be used to facilitate telemedicine visits and also connects with other devices to collect and report data. The solution offered by Catalia Health does not require the user to configure the robot in anyway, other than turn it on when they unbox the robot. As it is equipped with its own cellular modem, it aims to be more accessible to more patients, independently report data and provide 24/7 monitoring or as programmed.

Proteus Digital Health spent almost 20 years developing ingestible sensors and gained regulatory approval in 2017 for its "smart pill" from the FDA. The technology is incorporated into medications; a feat possible because the sensor employed was the size of a grain of sand and is coated on one side with copper and on the other with magnesium. When the pill is swallowed, gastric acid helps complete the circuit and generates a detectable, albeit tiny, electric current, which is detected by a sensor patch worn by the patient on their abdomen. This in turn connects with a mobile app and can be shared with those monitoring compliance. It helps complete a timestamp of when the medication was actually taken and so can determine adherence and compliance with a level of accuracy and granularity, which is hard to match for an oral ingestible medication which is self-administered. The patch is also a multimodal sensor and can measure activity and sleeping patterns, heart rate, and temperature. Some of the potential applications of the system included improving access to medications. Some payers and health systems will not provide some high-cost treatments to patients who are at risk of nonadherence. A pilot study examining this claim was performed and included 28 patients who were given treatment for hepatitis C that incorporated the smart pill technology. Of the 28 participants, 26 were cured and 94% of prescribed doses were taken (Bonacini et al., 2018). While this technology, its development, and the achievements of those who developed it and validated its utility are to be commended, it should also be noted that it may be used as a cautionary tale. At its pinnacle, Proteus Digital Health were valued at over $1.5 billion US dollars, and despite FDA approval of their technology in 2017, they were bankrupt by 2020, when their underlying assets including intellectual property were bought for $15 million US dollars by a pharmaceutical company who clearly understand the value proposition of the technology.

A multicenter randomized controlled trial of pelvic floor muscle training with a motion-based digital therapeutic device was performed versus pelvic floor muscle training alone for the treatment of stress-predominant urinary incontinence by a group of investigators from Massachusetts General Hospital, Northwestern University, the University of Oklahoma, Cedars Sinai, the Cleveland Clinic, Eastern Virginia Medical School, and the University of Alabama, and published in January 2022. They randomized 77 women but had to halt the trial early due to device technical considerations. However, before termination, those randomized to the intervention group installed a mobile application to their smartphone and paired with the device: Renovia Inc's leva digital therapeutic, which is an intravaginal insert equipped with accelerometers and which communicates wirelessly with the smartphone app. This in turn provides visual feedback to the patient. After 8 weeks, the primary outcomes, including change in Urinary Distress Inventory and the Patient Global Impression of Improvement, did not show any improvement between groups; however, the median number of stress urinary incontinence (SUI) episodes decreased from baseline by 1.7 per day in the intervention group compared to 0.7 in the control group, $P = .047$ (Weinstein, Dunivan, Guaderrama, & Richter, 2022).

A subsequent and larger prospective randomized controlled superiority trial, conducted remotely from September 2020 to March 2021, had 363 patients randomized to the same intervention as described in the earlier study by Weinstein et al. This larger subsequent study was powered to detect a difference in efficacy of pelvic floor training by using the levia digital therapeutic device with a home training program to reduce severity of symptoms and episodes of urinary incontinence. This trial demonstrated a significant reduction in both the median number of SUI episodes on the 3-day bladder diary (4 episode reduction vs. 3 episode reduction for the control group; $P = .005$) and also demonstrated significant improvements in both the UDI-6 score and PGI-I score (Weinstein, Collins, et al., 2022).

Digitally enabled treatments

As mentioned earlier in this chapter, there are many digitally enabled treatments focused at behavioral modification including weight loss and also chronic conditions such as diabetes which are of relevance to urology patients, but there are many more in various phases of development and, indeed, an entire world of possible digital therapeutics (and perhaps, also ailments) as the use of new technologies becomes more widespread. Treatments can be enabled by digital sensors, wearable devices, virtual reality headsets, and smart home devices. Helping a patient to adhere to a particular diet or fluid-intake schedule, or to pursue and continue a particular exercise routine or medication regimen can all be easily enabled through existing devices, software, and software as a service (SaaS) providers.

In late 2018, PEAR Therapeutics became the first company to have a mobile digital therapeutic, which significantly improved clinical outcomes in treatments for opioid use disorder, approved by the FDA (Federal Drug Administration, 2018). PEAR Therapeutics' prescription digital therapeutics use mobile applications as an adjunct to outpatient treatments for diseases in therapeutic areas such as psychiatric and neurological diseases. The app, called "reSET-O app", increases retention of patients in an outpatient treatment program and is a prescription cognitive behavioral therapy (CBT). While I was unable to locate a similar product in development for urology patients, the reSET-O app provides a clear roadmap for the improved care of a huge number of patients with urological conditions. CBT and other psychotherapeutic interventions have been demonstrated to improve the quality of life and reduce negative effects in patients with cancer: it can treat anxiety and depression as well as persistent fatigue and insomnia caused by prostate, bladder, or renal cancers (Gielissen, Verhagen, Witjes, & Bleijenberg, 2006; Johnson et al., 2016). CBT can also help as an adjunctive treatment for patients with sexual dysfunction (Shamseer et al., 2015). The impact of CBT on the quality of life in patients with prostate cancer was demonstrated by a randomized controlled trial where, after 10 weeks of cognitive behavioral stress management, awareness of disease, change of mood, and communication all significantly improved (Penedo et al., 2004). The realm of CBT is not limited to the 2.0 generation of devices. In November 2021, the first virtual reality digital therapeutic was approved by the FDA in the United States of America. The therapeutic called EaseVRx is an immersive virtually reality system that also uses CBT as well as other behavioral therapies to help with pain reduction in adults with chronic low back pain. The device allows provision of proven and effective "virtual care" to patients. The application of such innovations allows for gamification of therapy and encourages better compliance with treatment regimens. The uptake of virtual reality will likely increase as the cost of devices capable of creating or displaying ultrarealistic environments becomes attainable to more and more. The immersive experience in therapy is not dissimilar to the simulated environment used in urological training, where surgeons can learn how to act, react, and prepare for unfamiliar situations and ultimately gain mastery of them. Similarly, patients can prepare for how they might feel, or act, and prepare to learn about stoma care, for instance, before they wake up after surgery, experiencing the physiological trauma of radical surgery and under the residual effects of anesthesia and sedatives. These are very real concerns for patients and can help patients be more fully informed prior to various therapies and also help them prepare for their rehabilitation.

The use of AI in software treatments is driving personalization and increasing engagement. AI-enabled therapeutics can provide a diagnosis and/or truly personalize care by tailoring the treatment for that patient. It can also anticipate patient needs and challenges based on the individual's behavior. This allows for a much more efficient and effective care plan that can be updated as the individual's needs change. Much of the technology required is miniaturized and made sufficiently desirable, and includes functional devices to smartphones and watches, to digital personal assistants and wearable sensors. For example, Clickotine, a digital therapeutics platform helps smokers quit using customized plans and medically proven strategies to overcome cravings and also provide supports to cease using tobacco. The application also requires various device permissions, which allows it to not just track user behavior but make recommendations based on defined rules—for example, if the user had mentioned getting nicotine cravings when they would consume coffee or if in a bar, the app would provide a message of support to the user when they entered a geofenced area or they made a purchase of a coffee using their smart device. Again, while I was unable to find a company focused on patients with urological conditions, the technology and expertise exist and has manifested a functional and available application, which can help countless urology patients who may need to quit tobacco, reduce caffeine intake or who need to reduce fluid intake after a certain time.

Barriers to adoption

Digital therapeutics have demonstrated that they offer meaningful and significant solutions to disparate and often poorly addressed elements of healthcare. As alluded to above, digital therapeutics have yet to become mainstream, not just in urology but all of healthcare. This is due to multiple barriers which are currently retarding greater adoption.

Reimbursement for digital therapies is similar to most new adjunctive treatments, subject to the vagaries of payers and insurance companies. Each reserves the right to cover a therapy but, in general, demonstrating safety, efficacy and demonstrating utility in the at-risk group are the most basic of hurdles to be crossed. In general, if a digital therapy aims to replace another proven intervention, pharmaceutical or otherwise, the barriers are higher. But digital therapies that help monitor, or are adjunctive therapies, or those which complement or improve compliance or efficacy are often considered more palatable. As payment models across the globe are in flux and more advocate for outcomes-based pricing models, digital therapeutics may offer a very attractive proposition to developers of all sorts of therapeutics. They will not only offer a method to potentially augment other therapies, but also are well positioned to provide hard data on the impact on health-related quality of life, offering insights into improved patient function even before the patient's next scheduled visit. This, coupled with the relatively low development cost and relatively shorter development time, will help incentivize their development and incorporation into the treatment protocol for all novel therapies, pharmacological or otherwise.

There are hundreds of thousands of "apps" on various application marketplaces (including Android's Google Play Store, and Apple's App Store for iOS), which claim a health-related purpose. Consumers can become disillusioned or lack confidence in a legitimate application because they may first seek an application to help self-manage before they attend their physician. They may come to associate such applications as low value, or invasive, and may even be deterred by the somewhat extensive list of permissions that applications utilize—particularly those asking to access your storage, your contacts and messages, your location and GPS tracking settings, or those requesting network control and the ability to wake your device from sleep among others. While each of these may have a legitimate and benign purpose in a legitimate prescription digital therapeutic, patients who are also consumers of digital products may be wary and reluctant to share this information. The FDA requires all medical device companies to identify and mitigate cybersecurity risks as part of premarket submissions, but best practice standards are rapidly evolving (Celi, Miao, Arneson, Wang, & Butte, 2022).

The use of AI weaves in another layer of complexity, which may hinder the adoption of digital therapeutics employing such methods. There have been notable examples of the limitations of AI-derived tools to discriminate along the lines of data it was exposed to during its training: the data used in many training datasets, and in particular clinical data available for use in medicine, are often biased by those for whom data are available in an electronic format. This tends to favor those from western nations and those from areas where health systems have been using electronic medical records for longer. This could lead to biased decisions and inequitable delivery of healthcare. Some have proposed a checklist for AI models: as with regulatory labeling for other therapeutics, digital therapeutics employing AI and similar methods should include a labeling requirement that makes it clear how such algorithms and tools were trained, as well as clear descriptions of the cohort demographics and social determinants of health (Norgeot et al., 2020).

As with all novel devices, whether endoscopic, laparoscopic, robotic, or other disruptive innovations in medicine or industry, reluctance and resistance to change can be expected. Urologists are also well placed to help improve patient experience and the quality of life by acting as early adopters and vigilant gatekeepers for this next wave of innovation.

Bibliography

Adhikary, R., Kolwankar, S., Verma, R., Pawar, S., Agarwal, R., Naidu, B. M., ... Saboo, B. (2021). Abstract #997302: Real-world effectiveness of digital therapeutics towards achieving weight loss in people with obesity and metabolic syndrome. *Endocrine Practice, 27*(6), S77–S78. https://doi.org/10.1016/j.eprac.2021.04.633

Bal, K., Oder, M., Sahin, A. S., Karatas, C. T., Demir, O., Can, E., ... Esen, A. A. (2007). Prevalence of metabolic syndrome and its association with erectile dysfunction among urologic patients: Metabolic backgrounds of erectile dysfunction. *Urology, 69*(2), 356–360. https://doi.org/10.1016/j.urology.2006.09.057

Bonacini, M., Kim, Y., Pitney, C., McKoin, L., Tran, M., & Landis, C. (2018). 2220. Wirelessly observed therapy with a digital medicines program to optimize adherence and target interventions for oral hepatitis C treatment. *Open Forum Infectious Diseases, 5*(Suppl. 1_), S656. https://doi.org/10.1093/ofid/ofy210.1873

Celi, L. A., Miao, B. Y., Arneson, D., Wang, M., & Butte, A. J. (2022). Open challenges in developing digital therapeutics in the United States. *PLOS Digital Health, 1*(1). https://doi.org/10.1371/journal.pdig.0000008

Federal Drug Administration. (2018). *FDA clears mobile medical app to help those with opioid use disorder stay in recovery programs* [Press release]. Retrieved from https://www.fda.gov/news-events/press-announcements/fda-clears-mobile-medical-app-help-those-opioid-use-disorder-stay-recovery-programs.

Gielissen, M. F., Verhagen, S., Witjes, F., & Bleijenberg, G. (2006). Effects of cognitive behavior therapy in severely fatigued disease-free cancer patients compared with patients waiting for cognitive behavior therapy: A randomized controlled trial. *Journal of Clinical Oncology, 24*(30), 4882–4887. https://doi.org/10.1200/JCO.2006.06.8270

Jeong, Y. M., Lee, E., Kim, K. I., Chung, J. E., In Park, H., Lee, B. K., & Gwak, H. S. (2016). Association of pre-operative medication use with post-operative delirium in surgical oncology patients receiving comprehensive geriatric assessment. *BMC Geriatrics, 16*, 134. https://doi.org/10.1186/s12877-016-0311-5

Johnson, J. A., Rash, J. A., Campbell, T. S., Savard, J., Gehrman, P. R., Perlis, M., ... Garland, S. N. (2016). A systematic review and meta-analysis of randomized controlled trials of cognitive behavior therapy for insomnia (CBT-I) in cancer survivors. *Sleep Medicine Reviews, 27*, 20–28. https://doi.org/10.1016/j.smrv.2015.07.001

Norgeot, B., Quer, G., Beaulieu-Jones, B. K., Torkamani, A., Dias, R., Gianfrancesco, M., ... Butte, A. J. (2020). Minimum information about clinical artificial intelligence modeling: The MI-CLAIM checklist. *Nature Medicine, 26*(9), 1320–1324. https://doi.org/10.1038/s41591-020-1041-y

Penedo, F. J., Dahn, J. R., Molton, I., Gonzalez, J. S., Kinsinger, D., Roos, B. A., ... Antoni, M. H. (2004). Cognitive-behavioral stress management improves stress-management skills and quality of life in men recovering from treatment of prostate carcinoma. *Cancer, 100*(1), 192–200. https://doi.org/10.1002/cncr.11894

Schuster, M., Neumann, C., Neumann, K., Braun, J., Geldner, G., Martin, J., … Group, C. S. (2011). The effect of hospital size and surgical service on case cancellation in elective surgery: Results from a prospective multicenter study. *Anesthesia & Analgesia, 113*(3), 578–585. https://doi.org/10.1213/ANE.0b013e318222be4d

Shamseer, L., Moher, D., Clarke, M., Ghersi, D., Liberati, A., Petticrew, M., … Group, P.-P. (2015). Preferred reporting items for systematic review and meta-analysis protocols (PRISMA-P) 2015: Elaboration and explanation. *BMJ, 350*, g7647. https://doi.org/10.1136/bmj.g7647

Weinstein, M. M., Collins, S., Quiroz, L., Anger, J. T., Paraiso, M. F. R., DeLong, J., & Richter, H. E. (2022). Multicenter randomized controlled trial of pelvic floor muscle training with a motion-based digital therapeutic device versus pelvic floor muscle training alone for treatment of stress-predominant urinary incontinence. *Female Pelvic Medicine and Reconstructive Surgery, 28*(1), 1–6. https://doi.org/10.1097/SPV.0000000000001052

Weinstein, M. M., Dunivan, G., Guaderrama, N. M., & Richter, H. E. (2022). Digital therapeutic device for urinary incontinence: A randomized controlled trial. *Obstetrics and Gynecology, 139*(4), 606–615. https://doi.org/10.1097/AOG.0000000000004725

Remote surgery

10

Introduction

Urology is a long-established specialty, and many urologists still use surgical instruments such as urethral sounds, which have been in use since at least 3000 BC and not changed much in hundreds of years of practice. Urology is also a specialization which is highly technical and promotes innovation. Endoscopic and laparoscopic surgeries dominate urological practice and, by their nature, are well suited to innovation and the introduction of innovative techniques and technology. Unsurprisingly, urologists have been at the forefront of technological innovation in recent years; in particular, the adoption of robotic surgery. But the specialty and medical community, in general, need to be proactive in the scientific evaluation of new technologies and their further evolution (Murphy, Challacombe, Khan, & Dasgupta, 2006).

Remote surgery can encompass many things, from telementoring to telesurgery. Telesurgery, specifically, is operating through the use of a surgical robot, which is actively controlled by a distant operator, and it is only possible because of the development of robotic surgical systems. Over the past 20 years, robotic surgery has become a mainstay of hospital systems around the world. The da Vinci robotic system from Intuitive Surgical Inc. (Sunnyvale, CA, USA) is the global leader at present and has led this transformation. Thanks to its innovative technology and unique revenue model, Intuitive has installed over 6730 surgical robotic systems worldwide in this time period. The rapid adoption and spread of the surgical robot have been driven by many important industry-specific factors. There was a dramatic leap from open to robotic procedures in urology and, in terms of gradual technological adoption, laparoscopic surgeries were in some instances almost entirely leapfrogged by robot-assisted laparoscopic surgeries.

Between 1998 and 2011, the number of open radical prostatectomy procedures decreased by 70%, and 18% of hospitals in the United States stopped performing the procedure altogether (Tyson et al., 2016). One study which utilized the National Inpatient Sample database found that between 2008 and 2011, the number of laparoscopic radical prostatectomy procedures dropped by 90%. The rapid adoption and fast-forwarding of a process, which is often a gradual and incremental technological progress, is not new to the field of urology. Telehealth now has a recent and relevant precedent. And the barriers to future innovations in the delivery of care need not seem so insurmountable any more.

The history of urological surgery is full of the advances offered by urological devices, and this is still true of robotics. In the past two decades, da Vinci's intuitive systems have been market leaders. Intuitive continue to innovate with the development of the Si, X, Xi, and SP systems. Advances in robotics research and development are happening around the world in Korea, China, Japan, Ireland, Germany, the United Kingdom, and Canada, as well as continuing in the United States. It has already begun to make robots smaller and cheaper (Loughlin, 2021).

The next major challenge in robotic surgery will be the further development of telesurgery, telementoring, telesurgery, and telepresence. Not only is there a shortage of urologists in the United States, but also a poor distribution of urologists. According to the American Urological Association, 62% of counties in the USA have no practicing urologist and it has recognized the workforce shortage as a federal advocacy priority (Nam, Daignault-Newton, Kraft, & Herrel, 2021).

In the home of the world's largest economy, great disparities exist in access to healthcare, where race, ethnicity, first spoken language, and rural dwelling status may result in being undertreated for significant diseases (Lundon et al., 2020; Maganty et al., 2020). This misdistribution is likely to worsen as economic and social gaps widen, and as more and more of the population urbanizes. Telerobotics and telementoring are two strategies for providing modern robotic technology and expertise to underserved areas, and this needs to accelerate in the future. The next great leap may well be fully autonomous robotic surgery.

History of robotic surgery

The history of robotic surgery is firmly rooted in the evolution of laparoscopic surgery. In 1986, the development of the first video computer chip that enabled magnification and projection of images on television screens led to the worldwide adoption of laparoscopic surgery (Shah, Bandari, Pelzman, Davies, & Jacobs, 2021). This rapid emergence of laparoscopic procedures sparked interest in exploring the possibilities of remote laparoscopy, which eventually led to the development of the first robotic surgical systems.

Among the first was the Green Stanford Research Institute Telepresence Surgical System (GTSS), a multidisciplinary research collaboration that began in the 1980s and was led by Dr. Phillip Green of the Stanford Research Institute. Similar to today's "master—slave" robotic surgical systems, this system included a remote operating area, a surgical workstation, and a three-dimensional view of the operating area. While comparable to standard laparoscopic instruments, the Green Surgical System instruments retained only four degrees of freedom (3). In 1992, this research area gained further momentum when the US Defense Advanced Research Projects Agency (DARPA) envisioned a robotic telesurgical system that would allow surgeons to perform live operations remotely on the battlefield, and provided research funding (Satava, 2022). Through this DARPA-funded advanced biomedical technology program, the Automated Endoscopy System for Optimal Positioning (AESOP) was developed in 1993 by Computer Motion, Inc.

After Dr. Green and his team performed the first remote telesurgical procedure on an ex-vivo pig intestine in 1994, the concept sparked the interest of Dr. Frederic Moll, a general surgeon who had previously founded and sold two companies using laparoscopic instruments: Origin Medisystems and Endotherapeutics. Moll enlisted the help of electrical engineers Robert Younge and John Freund (also a Harvard MBA graduate), and in 1995 they successfully licensed the technologies from the Stanford Research Institute, International Business Machines Corporation, and Massachusetts Institute of Technology, forming Intuitive Surgical Devices, Inc (later changed to Intuitive Surgical, Inc.). In the spring of 1996, they modified the GTSS model to include EndoWrist articulated technology, which allowed seven-degree wrist movements to mimic the human wrist, setting Intuitive apart from its competitors.

Instead of focusing on telemedicine, Intuitive sought to use EndoWrist technology to facilitate the adoption of its technology. Over the next 3 years, Intuitive would continue to review and customize its robot, until they registered with the Securities and Exchange Commission in 1998. Their registration documents with the SEC specifically did not mention radical prostatectomy as one of the possible uses of da Vinci. By the year 2000 though, several groups reported using the da Vinci to perform robotic prostatectomy using EndoWrist technology, and in May 2001, the da Vinci Surgical System received Food and Drug Administration approval for prostate surgery. As of December 2021, Intuitive Surgical had installed 6730 da Vinci robotic surgical systems worldwide, with 4139 da Vinci systems installed in the United States (and with ~1000 being installed in the United States between 2018 and 2021). Intuitive no longer have a monopoly on robotic surgery, and it is hoped that more competition in this sphere will spur greater innovation, greater access to care and better outcomes for patients.

Less than a decade ago, Stryker (Kalamazoo, Michigan) acquired Mako Surgical and its MAKOplasty robotic-arm interactive robotic orthopedic system for knee and hip replacement. The system integrates preoperative computed tomography (CT) modeling and determines a safe surgical area, and tactile boundaries constrain the robotic arm. While the company is not focused on urological applications, their integration of imaging modalities into a robotic surgical platform is noteworthy and provides a framework for how this may be adopted and evolved for other applications.

Avatera, a joint venture between Avatera Medical (Jena, Germany) and Force Dimension (Nyon, Switzerland), has been in development since 2011 (https://www.avatera.eu/en/avatera-sistema). It operates as a "master—slave" system similar to the da Vinci Surgery System. It is an open console that uses microscope-like technology with 3D-HD resolution, forceps-like handles, seven degrees of freedom, and four robotic arms mounted on a single cart. Unique to Avatera is its disposable system which aims to reduce costs. After obtaining the CE certification in November 2019, Avatera acquired FORWARDttc in August 2020 to use its engineering experience on mechatronic systems to develop hardware and software for robotics. While the company state they have completed cadaveric trials, preclinical studies have yet to be published in peer reviewed journals.

Kawasaki and Sysmex have collaborated in forming Medicaroid in 2013 to develop Hinotori, a Japanese robotic surgical system. Kawasaki is one of the world's largest industrial robotics companies, and Japan manufactures >50% of the world's market share of industrial robots. Hinotori was developed by Medicaroid with a stated goal "to serve and assist humans, not to replace humans." Hinotori has eight degrees of freedom, easy docking, and a 3D-HD viewer claiming "more than full HD resolution". There are four robotic arms attached to the cart, and the surgeon wears polarized glasses using a semiopen console with a microscope-like ocular lens. The system received regulatory approval in Japan in August 2020 (Cisu, Crocerossa, Carbonara, Porpiglia, & Autorino, 2021).

CMR Surgical started the development of a portable and modular robotic system in 2014 which is named Versius. It is unique in its relatively small size—being just 38×38 cm—and is intended to be highly portable, not just between operating rooms but also between hospitals. It includes an open surgical console with 3D-HD technology, three individually cart-mounted robotic arms with seven degrees of freedom, and has the capability of allowing the surgeon to sit or stand. In 2019, Versius was first introduced in a clinical setting in Pune, India. Regulatory approval was received in Australia in February 2020 for use in general surgery, gynecologic surgery, and urology. CE marking has not yet been obtained for its use in Europe nor have regulators in the US approved the Versius system.

Ethicon, Johnson and Johnson's medical device company, created a joint venture with Verily (a life sciences organization within Google) and created Verb Surgical in 2015. This has been seen as a combination of the medical instrument expertise of Ethicon and the artificial intelligence and visualization expertise of Google. While there is limited information on the Verb robotic system, Ethicon acquired Auris Health in February 2019. Auris developed robotic diagnostic and surgical devices, which were first used in lung cancer. A working prototype of the Verb Surgical System was reported to have been shown to Google and Johnson and Johnson executives in December 2019, but little else has been released on the system since then.

Medtronic entered the space with Hugo. Medtronic is the world's largest medical device company by revenue and has been working on a robotic surgical system since it acquired MiroSurge as part of its Covidien acquisition in 2014. Hugo was unveiled by Medtronic in 2019 as a modular system, where the surgeon sits in an open console with 3D-HD glasses. Dublin-based Medtronic announced it had received CE Mark approval for urologic and gynaecologic procedures in October 2021 and on February 2nd, 2022, announced the first procedure using the Hugo RAS system was a robotic prostatectomy performed in Aalst Belgium. Trials to enable approval for use in the USA are ongoing.

The origins of robotic surgery and telesurgery were initially academic, with military or space applications spurring development. There now appears to have been a loss of focus on more down-to-earth applications for telesurgery in the past decade. The German Aerospace Center created MiroSurge. Used mainly in research, the minimally invasive telesurgery platform consists of three robots and is equipped with torque sensors to capture feedback from reaction forces of manipulated tissue. Stanford Research Institute (who went on to become Intuitive Surgical) had a system named M7, which was part of the NASA Extreme Mission Operations (NEEMO) project, which included remote surgeries being performed under the sea as well as completing a surgical demonstration on a zero-gravity flight in 2007. Much of this foundational work has now been subsumed by the growing robotic surgery industrial complex, where the focus has been on providing services to the many. Now the technology has evolved and patents on foundational work no longer restrict access to resource-limited healthcare systems, the needs of patients and remote communities need to take center stage once more.

Telementoring

The use of videoconferencing to support physicians overseas or in areas with increased needs or limited resources is not new. Médecins Sans Frontières uses secure videoconferencing for clinical case reviews, clinical supervision, patient consultations, and training. During the COVID-19 pandemic, surgeons became more comfortable using telepresence platforms to collaborate with colleagues. The proliferation of videoconferencing and its ability to support geographically-dispersed teams means that remote teaching and learning could play a greater role in surgical training and practice, both nationally and internationally (Best, 2022).

Several new digital platforms aim to build on traditional video conferencing, from the provision of verbal guidance in real time to telestration, allowing the distant surgeon to provide visual aides to the operating surgeon. This allows surgeons to collaborate on cases in real time with features that replicate in-person mentoring as occurs in real-world practice. One such example is Proximie, which combines video conferencing with technologies like augmented reality and allows surgeons in one location to see multiple views of an operating room in another location.

Such systems mean you can tag, outline, label and otherwise interact with the operative field of view and make real-time contributions as the case progresses. A project is underway in Makueni County, Kenya, to use this technology to improve the safety of caesarean sections. The district, which has a population of more than 900,000, has just three obstetricians and gynecologists working in two hospitals, with most caesarean sections performed by general practitioners or doctors performing compulsory service after graduation. As part of the Obstetric Safe Surgery project, supported by organizations such as Jhpiego, affiliated with John Hopkins University in the USA, Proximie technology has been implemented in five hospitals in the province with the aim of improving maternal and neonatal outcomes. Using technology, consultants guide medical officers through simulated caesarean sections, as well as training courses on infection prevention, use of the World Health Organization surgical safety checklist, administration of anesthesia, and infant care. More experienced healthcare providers are also beginning to remotely assist on elective cases, with Proximie using four theater views—the entire theater, surgical site, anesthesia, and child's CPR room—to provide an overview of the surgery. Surgeons can remotely annotate and highlight parts of the operating field for those in the room and be guided through the procedure by their remote proctor/mentor (Best, 2022).

Intuitive Surgical also have a software solution that supports telestration, which is called Connect and is integrated into their da Vinci Surgical System. The mentor can offer verbal and video-aided guidance overlaying the surgeon's field of view directly within the surgeon console, so the operating surgeon does not need a separate video input (Shin et al., 2015).

Telesurgery

Remote collaboration technology is evolving to the point where surgeons in one location can use surgical robots to operate on patients in another location. A handful of such remote operations has already been performed on cadavers, animal and human models.

Operation Lindbergh was the first transcontinental telesurgical operation ever performed: In 2001, Jacques Marescaux performed a laparoscopic cholecystectomy on a 68-year-old lady in Strasbourg, France, using a ZEUS robotic system positioned in Mount Sinai Hospital in New York, USA. The procedure was performed without complication, and the patient was discharged successfully 48 hours later (Raison, Khan, & Challacombe, 2015). Other pioneering work includes the report of the insertion of a deep brain stimulator into a patient with Parkinson's disease by a surgeon controlling a robotic arm from a city almost 3000 km away.

One of the few randomized controlled trials assessing telesurgery involved percutaneous access to the kidney and comparing human and robotic percutaneous renal access (Challacombe et al., 2005). This groundbreaking study demonstrated the feasibility of remote transatlantic surgery using robots that operate with comparable efficiency and efficacy when controlled at distances of, as the others have stated, "5 meters or 5000 miles" (Raison et al., 2015). However, despite such resounding early successes, the further development and promulgation of telesurgery has been disappointingly slow.

World's first telesurgery service

St. Joseph's Hospital in Hamilton, Canada and North Bay General Hospital, 400 km north of Hamilton, are the sites of the world's first telesurgery service. It was established on February 28, 2003, and at the time, the service utilized a Zeus-TS surgical system in North Bay and a 15 Mbps commercially available internet connection. This was a combination of telementoring and tele-assisted surgery.

Local North Bay surgeons and laparoscopic nurses were trained in the use of the robotic surgical system and devices before initiation of the telesurgery service.

Experienced technicians also attended each case to ensure smooth setup of the surgical arms. Meanwhile in Hamilton, the room from which the robotic surgeons work was equipped with two large screen televisions that displayed images from the North Bay operating room as well as the laparoscopic view. The sound of the North Bay operating room and the voices of the surgeon and laparoscopic staff could be heard through the loudspeakers. The environment was created so that the telerobotic surgeon could be immersed in the atmosphere of the North Bay operating room. The two surgeons also communicated constantly using wireless headphones.

Considerations on licensing and malpractice insurance for the "telesurgeon"

This pioneering work in telesurgery also draws attention to local, national, and international credentialing issues that may prove challenging. In the case of this service in Canada, all surgeons were medically insured by the Canadian Medical Protection Association. This is something which may be challenging if the service is offered across state or national boundaries, and similarly for medical licensing and credentialing. The service in Canada occurred because all staff had privileges at the hospital to perform advanced laparoscopic procedures. That, and a legal agreement between the surgeons and partners including both hospitals, the telecommunications company, the surgical system, and computer networking provider had been signed prior to the service initiating, where the scope of each party's responsibility during telerobotic surgical cases was defined. This is no simple undertaking, and the team who made the world's first telerobotic surgical service a reality deserve great commendation and recognition for not just pioneering this practice, but doing so in a clearly defined and collaborative manner. Their clearly defined protocols and procedures also act as a playbook, which enable further future services to build on their work.

Challenges for telesurgery

The spread of telesurgery will depend on the availability and access to two key technologies: surgical robotics and reliable, stable high-speed internet access. While we have discussed some of the encouraging innovation in surgical robotics, internet access is synonymous in some realms with a basic utility and unfortunately, like many other basic utilities, it is not as ubiquitously available or reliable as it need be. This may be in part due to the huge demands for this utility.

Many advocate for the greater availability of 5G networks as a solution to provide access to reliable and stable high-speed internet access. However, the question as to its suitability received an answer of sorts when the European Commission and the European Agency for Cybersecurity published a report warning of serious security concerns (Robles-Carrillo, 2021). Regardless of any political or strategic policies of national interest, the technological and infrastructural advantages of 5G mean it is currently not the solution that telesurgery has sought. 5G wavelengths are in the order of millimeters, and their range is currently approximately 1000 ft. As such, to maintain a reliable signal and maintain the benefits of high speed, high bandwidth, and lower latency, each cell tower needs to have another 5G tower in similarly close proximity, or there needs to be a cabled connection to that tower. Either way, the 5G tower remains a bandwidth bottleneck, where the capacity of 5G is currently dwarfed by the capacity of a cabled connection, and 5G really doesn't even offer "last mile" connectivity, but rather last 1000 feet connectivity. In addition, 5G competes for spectrum bands, which is becoming ever more competitive, and is discussed in more detail elsewhere in this book.

Not to detract from 5G, where speeds can range from 50 Mbit/s to the fastest of 4000 Mbit/s ($\sim$4 Gigabits per second), fiber cables such as those used by Facebook can currently carry 13 Tpbs (more than 3000 $\times$ more), and a recent experiment by Facebook and Nokia Bell labs suggests that the fibers could carry 32 Tbps. The issue that fast and reliable internet needs to solve for in telesurgery is rural, remote, and difficult to access areas. If the distance that 5G can jump is less than one mile, then it's not even the right technology to be discussing for telesurgery (Farroha, 2019).

Meanwhile satellite internet providers have proven their worth in this realm, where government bodies such as militaries use dedicated satellites for event critical missions, and where no bandwidth is shared and latency is minimal. There is much development in this space and tech companies like Viasat and Starlink may accelerate access to such technology, and others promise greater technological innovation in this field.

Such mobile networks reduce latency—the delay between sending and receiving data—to less than 1 millisecond. At the same time, it will increase the download speed to a theoretical peak of over 1 gigabit per second. Both are significant steps forward from what is currently available on 4G networks and are needed to allow the surgeon and robot to work in such an environment in real time, with no delay between the surgeon and robot's movements.

A significant cause of latency results from the compression—decompression or encoding and decoding of high-quality video into a digital signal for transmission. A mathematical integration exists, where the degree of compression affects the size of the video, and hence the transmission time of the video from origin to destination. Almost all studies and publications describing telementoring or telesurgery suggest software is used for video compression—decompression. Groups have even implemented a form of machine learning to aide in further reducing file size whereby they sacrifice video resolution, allowing an algorithm to make the executive decision on where the focus of attention should be and encoding a portion of the video in high quality with the background region in low quality (Hassan, Ghafoor, Tariq, Zia, & Ahmad, 2019). This great effort could overshadow more practical and indeed higher-quality solutions that already exist. The transmission of live video is not a new problem, and certainly not one that only telesurgery requires a solution for. Everyone from military and government intelligence services to live news networks and social media websites have a need for a solution to this problem. And indeed, most have used hardware solutions which provide far superior latency times and compression–decompression times than any software solution is capable of achieving. In fact, an entire industry exists for this one challenge, and superior solutions exist, albeit at a cost. For example, NETINT offers a commercially available hardware AV1 encoder for data centers, utilizing Codensity G5 video transcoders, and allows and enables up to 7680 FPS at 4K broadcast quality video, but with ultra-low latency performance that makes step function improvements in video transmission. Hardware encoding for telesurgery should be the current default method used as it doesn't require sacrificing video quality for latency time.

Conclusion

Telerobotic remote surgery is already in routine use, and published data demonstrate that high-quality surgical services are possible across continents and through an already established telesurgical program offered to patients in rural communities. The hope remains that broader adoption of telesurgery will allow hospitals in remote or poor areas to access surgeons from elsewhere to perform surgeries. Technology currently available is such that there is little in the way but societal and political will to deliver such care right now.

Bibliography

Best, J. (2022). From Ukraine to remote robotics: How videoconferencing and next generation technology are transforming surgery. *British Medical Journal, 377,* o1078. https://doi.org/10.1136/bmj.o1078

Challacombe, B., Patriciu, A., Glass, J., Aron, M., Jarrett, T., Kim, F., … Dasgupta, P. (2005). A randomized controlled trial of human versus robotic and telerobotic access to the kidney as the first step in percutaneous nephrolithotomy. *Randomized Controlled Trial, 10*(3), 165–171.

Cisu, T., Crocerossa, F., Carbonara, U., Porpiglia, F., & Autorino, R. (2021). New robotic surgical systems in urology: An update. *Current Opinion in Urology, 31*(1), 37–42. https://doi.org/10.1097/MOU.0000000000000833

Farroha, J. S.,F. B. S. (2019). Enabling intelligent battlefield healthcare through secure cyber medicine. *Open Architecture/Open Business Model Net-Centric Systems and Defense Transformation.* https://doi.org/10.1117/12.2516021

Hassan, A., Ghafoor, M., Tariq, S. A., Zia, T., & Ahmad, W. (2019). High efficiency video coding (HEVC)-Based surgical telementoring system using shallow convolutional neural network. *Journal of Digital Imaging, 32*(6), 1027–1043. https://doi.org/10.1007/s10278-019-00206-2

Loughlin, K. R. (2021). Forward: Robotic urology: Remember the future. *Urology Clinics of North America, 48*(1). https://doi.org/10.1016/j.ucl.2020.10.001. xiii-xiv.

Lundon, D. J., Mohamed, N., Lantz, A., Goltz, H. H., Kelly, B. D., & Tewari, A. K. (2020). Social determinants predict outcomes in data from a multi-ethnic cohort of 20,899 patients investigated for COVID-19. *Front Public Health, 8,* 571364. https://doi.org/10.3389/fpubh.2020.571364

Maganty, A., Sabik, L. M., Sun, Z., Eom, K. Y., Li, J., Davies, B. J., & Jacobs, B. L. (2020). Under treatment of prostate cancer in rural locations. *The Journal of Urology, 203*(1), 108–114. https://doi.org/10.1097/JU.0000000000000500

Murphy, D., Challacombe, B., Khan, M. S., & Dasgupta, P. (2006). Robotic technology in urology. *Postgraduate Medical Journal, 82*(973), 743–747. https://doi.org/10.1136/pgmj.2006.048140

Nam, C. S., Daignault-Newton, S., Kraft, K. H., & Herrel, L. A. (2021). Projected US urology workforce per capita, 2020-2060. *JAMA Network Open, 4*(11), e2133864. https://doi.org/10.1001/jamanetworkopen.2021.33864

Raison, N., Khan, M. S., & Challacombe, B. (2015). Telemedicine in surgery: What are the opportunities and hurdles to realising the potential? *Current Urology Report, 16*(7), 43. https://doi.org/10.1007/s11934-015-0522-x

Robles-Carrillo, M. (2021). European Union policy on 5G: Context, scope and limits. *Telecommunications Policy, 45*(8). https://doi.org/10.1016/j.telpol.2021.102216

Satava, R. M. (2022). Surgical robotics: the early chronicles: a personal historical perspective. *Surg Laparoscopy Endoscopy & Percutaneous Techniques, 12*(1), 6–16. https://doi.org/10.1097/00129689-200202000-00002

Shah, A. A., Bandari, J., Pelzman, D., Davies, B. J., & Jacobs, B. L. (2021). Diffusion and adoption of the surgical robot in urology. *Translational Andrology and Urology, 10*(5), 2151–2157. https://doi.org/10.21037/tau.2019.11.33

Shin, D. H., Dalag, L., Azhar, R. A., Santomauro, M., Satkunasivam, R., Metcalfe, C., ... Hung, A. J. (2015). A novel interface for the telementoring of robotic surgery. *BJU International, 116*(2), 302–308. https://doi.org/10.1111/bju.12985

Tyson, M. D., 2nd, Andrews, P. E., Ferrigni, R. F., Humphreys, M. R., Parker, A. S., & Castle, E. P. (2016). Radical prostatectomy trends in the United States: 1998 to 2011. *Mayo Clinic Proceedings, 91*(1), 10–16. https://doi.org/10.1016/j.mayocp.2015.09.018

E-prescribing

11

Introduction

Electronic prescribing or e-prescribing has been identified as an important technology and stepping stone for improving the safety, quality, and efficiency of healthcare (Grossman, Gerland, Reed, & Fahlman, 2007). E-prescribing was initially touted as the "killer app" that would lead to wider adoption of e-health and telehealth by physicians, especially in small practices. The difference between what most would have envisaged and what is the current reality in most states and nations, points at design and operational failure. One feature touted over a decade ago was the ability to maintain a complete medication list, and a recent medication history for each patient; complete with decision support tools which would alert and remind prescribers and those dispensing of any relevant information such as contraindications, interactions, and dosing issues. If one were completing a checklist, each of these items could be said to have been provided. However a patient attending one healthcare provider doesn't necessarily have access to the same records or even the full record of dispensed drugs that another provider, in another health system has. It is also the case that different provider locations, within the same health systems, but that utilizes different electronic health records (EHR), sometimes do not have a common, unified and complete record of prescribed and dispensed drugs. Similarly, outside of some states enacting legislation covering the need to maintain a centralized record of dispensation of controlled substances, most pharmacies cannot be certain that they have a complete record of all the drugs a given patient has been dispensed, as patients may use any number of competing chain, independent, online, or specialty pharmacies, and there is no centralized record of care.

In retrospect, while e-prescribing adoption did increase in the past decade, most of the credit for its uptake should be attributed to Medicare and Medicaid EHR incentive programs, which began circa 2010 in the United States (Fig. 11.1). The promises that e-prescribing systems would increase patient safety and reduce costs through improved legibility and improved practice efficiency were not fully realized. While practice administrators may no longer have to direct calls from pharmacies unable to decipher a handwritten prescription, and healthcare providers may not have to have their work interrupted over their handwriting, they still need to confirm the intended drug, its dose or route of administration, are correct. While less

Telehealth in Urology. https://doi.org/10.1016/B978-0-323-87480-9.00001-4

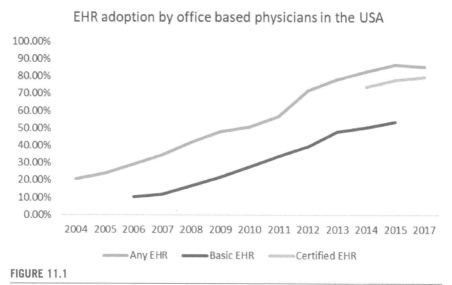

FIGURE 11.1

Electronic Health Record adoption by office-based physicians in the United States of America.

Source: HealthIT.gov

interruptions to work may have occurred, the promise of improved patient safety should really have been the only priority. E-prescriptions in many respects reduced the barrier to access to medicines, including controlled and addictive medicines. However, e-prescribing systems have and continue to experience many issues hampering realization of their potential (Abramson, Patel, Pfoh, & Kaushal, 2016).

Reducing barriers to access to prescription drugs is very clearly a two-edged sword. Legislation in the United States has been introduced by states to attempt to improve patient safety, reduce error rates in prescribing, and reduce the occurrence of prescription fraud. For example, while overall opioid prescribing rates decline in the United States of America following the opioid epidemic, e-prescriptions for opioids increased by more than a third (Achar, Sinha, & Norcross, 2021). New York State, for example, passed a law in March 2016 mandating healthcare providers to issue e-prescriptions for controlled substances in Schedules II through V, with only some exceptions. Yet there is no evidence to suggest that these initiatives have done anything to reduce abuse of controlled substances other than to track legitimately prescribed opioids. Ultimately, the gatekeeper to the legal access of controlled and addictive substances such as these, is the prescribing physician. While technology may promise improved legibility and a digital prompt to remind the prescriber of spelling and dose, it may also facilitate the abuse of an already overworked and underresourced healthcare staff. There is concern that the ease of e-prescription may be a tempting short-term solution, but not necessarily be the optimal mode of care.

E-prescribing—a tool to address the large burden of urological disease and the limited workforce?

The burden of urological disease in America is immense, both financially and individually (Lydia Feinstein, 2018). Societies such as the American Urological Association have done much to highlight the need for greater access to care, and also advocated to increase the number of specialists to treat patients and address disparities in access. Despite such efforts, poor access to care and an overburdened system among other factors, has resulted in many patients receiving shorter visits with caregivers (Hall, Link, Hu, Eggers, & McKinlay, 2009).

Many urological symptoms and conditions are responsive to medical therapy, such as lower urinary tract symptoms resulting from bladder outlet obstruction, overactive bladder and urinary incontinence, as well as erectile dysfunction. While not all of these conditions are universally cured by such interventions, many do obtain symptom relief and practice guidelines from various specialty interest groups, do include pharmacotherapies as a first-line care for some of these conditions. Some patients could be managed remotely, and at least for a period of time, without the need for in-person care.

The healthcare industry has traditionally relied on face-to-face consultations, where doctors hear and examine the patient, and can get a sense of what ills the patient. One of the most widely used interventions used to prevent and treat disease are pharmaceuticals. As a result, medicines are now one of the largest health expenditures, accounting for an average of 16% of total health expenditure in the Organisation for Economic Co-operation and Development (OECD) countries in 2015.

This is nowhere better demonstrated than by the growth of "digital health"/ "direct-to-consumer" providers such as those discussed elsewhere in this book, and discussed in a case example later in this chapter. Some of such providers consider medical conditions as "verticals" and have in many respects, "productified" ICD-10 codes. Profitable conditions where limited physician interaction can result in a prescription for an otherwise young and most often medication-free individual, now have multiple online companies, vying to on-board them, to a subscription service, which offers repeat prescriptions with minimal clinical review and oversight. It is an important distinction to make that these are businesses and not medical practices. While they often have the oversight of a medical director and employ (most often as contractors), physician assistants/physician associates or nurse specialists, many are public companies, and all that the author is aware of are for profit entities. In one respect, these businesses improve access to "care." However, it could be argued that such businesses only provide access to the sort of care that is a monetizable model of recurrent prescriptions, often fulfilled by the company themselves, using their own branded generic medication, and charging a healthy markup above generic costs, which would be available to patients accessing care through a conventional healthcare setting such as their urologist. It has been said these businesses are competing to medicate young and healthy individuals for conditions, which often are complex and that would benefit most from multidisciplinary care. There is no doubt though that making healthcare a consumer product, infinite and on-demand, diminishes the importance of the patient—physician relationship, and disempowers healthcare providers as health advocates. Without that central relationship, providers can no longer fully advocate for their patients and indeed really don't have patients any longer, so much as tasks to complete in a work queue.

Opportunities for e-prescribing

The third largest category of healthcare spending across the OECD is for medical goods. On average (see Fig. 11.2), the proportion of spending by category including medical goods (under which pharmaceuticals and other prescription goods are included) has remained stable over this time period. Price differences for international goods such as medicines tend to vary less across countries than for locally produced services (such as care provision). As a result, in low-income countries, spending on medical goods (including prescribed medicines) often accounts for a higher share of health spending than spending on services. Consequently, expenditure on medical goods accounted for almost a third of all healthcare expenditure in

Health Expenditure by type of service across 31 OECD nations

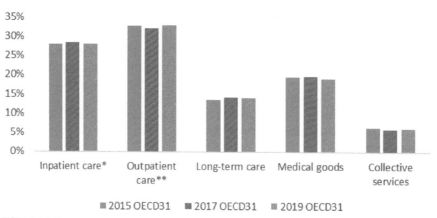

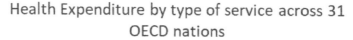
■ 2015 OECD31   ■ 2017 OECD31   ■ 2019 OECD31

FIGURE 11.2

Health expenditure by type of service across 31 OECD nations has remained stable on aggregate over the period including 2015, 2017, and 2019.
*Refers to curative-rehabilitative care in inpatient and day care settings. **Includes home care and ancillary services.

Sources: OECD Health Statistics, 2017, 2019 and 2021 reports.

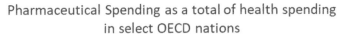

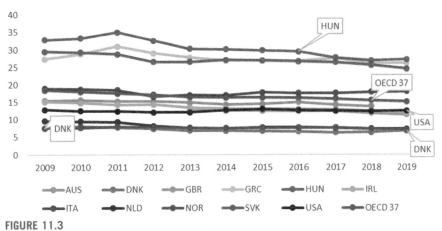

FIGURE 11.3

Pharmaceutical spending as a total of health spending in select OECD nations, and an average figure for 37 OECD nations, between the years 2009 and 2019.

Sources: OECD Health Statistics.

Hungary and the Slovak Republic in 2019. In Denmark, Norway, and the Netherlands, on the other hand, the shares were much lower with about 10% of total health expenditure (see Fig.11.3).

Drug misuse and diversion in urology is not a new problem

Prescription drug diversion is defined as the unlawful channeling of regulated pharmaceuticals from legal sources to the illicit marketplace. This includes transferring drugs to people they were not prescribed for. There are a number of scheduled and controlled substances commonly prescribed by urologists (see Table 11.1).

A recent study of opioid prescription patterns in patients undergoing urological surgery noted that >21% were preoperative users of opioids, and unsurprisingly that amid an opioid epidemic in the United States, that those already using opioids preprocedure were significantly more likely to get a prescription refill than those who were opioid naïve, where rates were 23.4% versus 11.3%, respectively, in a study of over 11,000 patients (Ziegelmann et al., 2019). It is also notable that in this same study, 78% were prescribed an opioid at discharge, and the subgroup of patients with the highest rate of refilling their opioid prescription, out of a cohort of patients including open cystoprostatectomy patients with ileal conduit/ileal neobladder, were the patients who underwent ureteral stent placement, where 25.9% obtained a refill on their prescription for opioids.

Table 11.1 Categories of drugs in the United States Controlled Substances Act and examples which may be prescribed by urologists.

Schedule	Abuse potential	Dependence	Approved medical use	Examples
I	High	May lead to psychological or physical dependence	No	–
II	High	May lead to severe psychological or physical dependence	Yes	Oxycodone morphine Codeine
III	< than schedule I and II	Moderate to low physical dependence or high psychological dependence	Yes	Anabolic steroids like testosterone Tylenol with codeine
IV	Low	May lead to psychological or physical dependence	Yes	Benzodiazepines like diazepam, alprazolam, lorazepam
V	Low	May lead to psychological or physical dependence	Yes	Gabapentin and pregabalin (in some states) Cough preparations containing low concentrations of codeine

For opioids, diversion has been shown to be proportional to the number of prescriptions written without supervised use (Bell, 2010). While it is difficult to quantify the extent to which prescriptions provided by urologists are diverted or abused, opioid prescriptions following urological procedures in the United States of America remain common, despite being amidst what has publicly been declared an opioid epidemic. Many have identified "overprescription" of narcotics in urological practice, and the urological literature has described it for over a decade, and yet the practice persists (Bates, Laciak, Southwick, & Bishoff, 2011; Ziegelmann et al., 2019). It is not uncommon for drug prescriptions provided on hospital discharge to be used to influence ongoing prescribing by other physicians, such as general practitioners or other specialists, if the patient seeks further medical care at a later time (Wood, 2015).

There has also been an ongoing increase in the year-over-year volume of testosterone prescriptions. Notable among the Food and Drug Administration (FDA) data on testosterone prescriptions in the United States of America, is that 13% of prescriptions were to men younger than 40 years of age, and men aged 40–60 years accounted for 70% (Gabrielsen, Najari, Alukal, & Eisenberg, 2016). The FDA figures paint a more conservative picture than data from a multicenter study from the Chicago metropolitan area, where 27% of new testosterone prescriptions (in 2012) were to men younger than 40 years of age (Malik, Wang, Lapin, Lakeman, & Helfand, 2015). This is relevant as the use of testosterone supplementation therapy in reproductive age men is generally not recommended by any society, particularly if the impact on fertility is not discussed with the patient, as exogenous testosterone supplementation effectively induces oligospermia and azoospermia in healthy men (Gu et al., 2009; Nieschlag et al., 2011).

Also notable from the multicenter study in the Chicago metropolitan area was that 29% of men tested and treated with testosterone replacement therapy had total serum testosterone levels >300 ng/dL, or what are considered by many as physiologically normal levels. While there are multiple guidelines on the diagnosis and management of hypogonadism, a relatively consistent recommendation is that testosterone only be prescribed to symptomatic patients, in whom low serum testosterone is documented on two independent and appropriately obtained laboratory tests, as well as ongoing monitoring of serum testosterone levels. Studies from the United States of America and United Kingdom have demonstrated a similar pattern where upwards of 87% did not have two tests prior to initiating testosterone, and upwards of 40% did not have any test performed prior to starting testosterone supplementation (Gabrielsen et al., 2016). The FDA included a label update to explicitly state men should have two separate morning serum testosterone values that are less than the normal range, before initiating testosterone supplementation, to the dose and administration section of the approved drug label.

These are ongoing concerns, and regardless of any touted safeguards which e-prescribing platforms may claim to have, pharmacovigilance, diligence regarding overtreatment, inappropriate treatment, and other such prescription patterns which can enable drug abuse and drug diversion, should be front of mind for all involved in e-prescribing to ensure patient safety and optimal care.

Challenges to e-prescribing

A study conducted between November 2005 and March 2006 of individuals from 26 organizations in the United States of America with e-prescribing and six without, included medical staff, practice administrators, and IT staff, and asked about e-prescribing. The study identified a number of opportunities and challenges, which persist to modern day (Grossman et al., 2007). Some of its main findings are summarized below, and while over 15 years old, most of the findings are still relevant today.

Maintaining complete medication lists

At the time of the study by Grossman et al. none of the respondents were able to access a comprehensive list of their patient's medications. Physicians at this time relied on patients as the main source of information on medications and doses taken.

Entering patient medication lists into an electronic medical record (EMR)/EHR or e-prescribing system is a major undertaking. Data must be at first entered manually but also then verified, which also requires in-person effort. At the time of this study, (and indeed it appears that this is still an ongoing issue), many physicians and practices do not keep up-to-date and complete medication lists.

Some e-prescribing systems can give access to medication histories by way of dispensed medications. However, pharmacy benefit managers (PBMs) in the United States often act as the middleman in this transaction, and so only PBMs that offer interconnectivity to their platform will be available. Similarly, PBMs by their nature only see purpose to be connected to pharmacies that fall under their plan. Prescriptions that do not utilize insurance or other health benefits will not be captured. Such systems also are imperfect at matching patients. As there is no universal patient identifier, such systems often use an algorithm including patient name and date of birth to match the patient in question, with existing prescription data. However, typographical and other errors often result in failed matches or only some of a patient's previous prescription data. Other limitations of such systems are that they do not indicate if a prescription has been discontinued.

Limited use of clinical decision support

Clinical decision support systems for e-prescribing ranges from basic features from name, form, strength, and duration assistance as well as alerts for drug–drug interactions, to drug allergies and contraindicated drugs, to more advanced features integrating lab result alerts for drug prescriptions to pharmacogenomics helping identify optimal drug choice and dosing, and automatic examination of drug records when a new allergy or symptom consistent with drug sensitivity or allergy is entered. Additional features such as notification when a prescription is not filled or refilled in a timely manner, and other behaviors of relevance to treatment compliance, to prompts for follow on laboratory tests to monitor drug levels or possible adverse events are also useful features that a clinical decision support system could offer as a feature of e-prescribing.

Of course, while many EMR/EHR systems offer such features, most users are unaware that they are available. Key to all such features is thorough engagement with the e-prescription/EMR system. If patient-specific information such as medication lists, allergies, and medical conditions are not recorded, and then kept up to date, then these features are of limited utility.

Most providers are familiar with the pop-up notifications for interaction alerts when prescribing a medication, and while important and particularly when prescribing a medication which the provider may not be familiar with, physicians very often override these alerts, and some even disable them altogether. Pop-up and notification fatigue is a real phenomenon amongst EMR users, and finding the right balance requires more active engagement at a practice level.

Obtaining accurate patient-specific formulary information

This is more relevant to jurisdictions where a patient's health insurer or provider offering financial assistance for medication costs has a preferred formulary. In such instances, certain treatments may only be available for patients; if other therapies have been tried, or perhaps only certain formulations or manufacturers will be covered by the insurer, and so the prescription must reflect this. While in theory, an e-prescribing platform is the perfect solution for such potentially burdensome work, it again requires accurate and up-to-date electronic records, coded and dated accurately. It can also require the entry of additional insurance information that may not be routinely collected—for example, a urology clinic may routinely collect health insurance information for services rendered, but some patients may receive their drug benefits from a different plan, and this is not always apparent and would require additional data entry by clinic staff.

It has also been noted that some e-prescribing systems omit formularies of major health insurers, as was the case for Medicaid being excluded from such a system. There have been longstanding problems with such systems and trust in the reliability of formulary data is poor, and combines poorly with frustrations over what a PBM thinks is an appropriate therapy for their members, versus what a physician or provider prescribes as the most medically appropriate drug therapy for the patient in front of them. Such is the nature of some healthcare systems, that the implementation of technological solutions requiring logic, seems to add further complexity, because of the seemingly illogical nature of the healthcare system.

Case examples—sexual health & erectile dysfunction

The European Society for Sexual Medicine has found that patient privacy and stigma concerns make e-medicine particularly useful (Kirana et al., 2020). Many men are ashamed of their sexual dysfunction and therefore do not seek medical help in a traditional form. Additionally, men avoid the urologist's office because of the invasive and uncomfortable physical exams (Brimley et al., 2021). A number of tech startups, perhaps naively categorized as telehealth providers currently address just this concern. Without focusing on any one company, the general workflow, similar if not common to most providers will be discussed. The predominant service offered under the banner of sexual health on such platforms is prescription of medications normally indicated for erectile dysfunction. While some offer services such as testing for some sexually transmitted infections (but not all), there is a notable absence of physician-led services for treatment, counseling, and contact tracing.

The International Index of Erectile Function (IIEF-5), a self-administered and validated questionnaire is often used as a web form to diagnose patients. Following completion of this questionnaire, users of such platforms are often informed that they are suitable or not to receive prescription therapy for their self-reported erectile dysfunction. The IIEF-5 is a widely accepted instrument, and the scoring and interpretation of the questionnaire is widely available, where lower IIEF-5 scores indicate poorer erectile function, and ranges from 5 to 25. Others have classified the use of such instruments by such online platforms, as "cursory self-diagnosis" and "normalization of erectile dysfunction as a lifestyle condition" (Shahinyan et al., 2020).

A recent study of men ≤ 40 years of age, being evaluated for erectile dysfunction, identified significant comorbidities in the study cohort that are not identified or managed by such online direct to consumer platforms. Such abnormalities included 40% of subjects having an abnormality on semen analysis, 35% having a varicocele on clinical examination, 54% having elevated low-density lipoprotein >100 mg/dL, 20% with a HbA1c $>5\%$, 11% with a follicle-stimulating hormone >7.5 miU/mL, and 20% had a total testosterone <300 ng/dL (Shahinyan et al., 2020). The authors of this study discussed the subscription format of these platforms that results in men ending up as chronic users of PDE-5 inhibitors without adequate follow-up or reevaluation, and how that contrasts with typical office-based urology evaluation and treatment with interval follow-ups; as in their cohort of men ≤ 40 years attending their clinic, they also provided counseling on lifestyle and risk factor modification and arranged reassessment after 3 months to evaluate effectiveness, and where PDE-5i therapy was titrated or discontinued based on patient's response. While it is apparent that the authors, and indeed all involved in urological care, are being accused of bias when commenting on such direct-to-consumer models which provide prescription medications, it is also clear, that such models as they currently exist, do not operate in accordance with guidance from expert groups, and typically overlook critical pathology, and ignore a critical opportunity for meaningful health interventions.

Sildenafil is already a medication which can be obtained without prescription, over-the-counter, in many countries, and other PDE-5i are or soon will be. Traditionally, over-the-counter prescription drugs have been limited to treating the symptoms of self-limiting minor medical conditions which, given their widespread availability, are easily diagnosed and have low potential for harm and abuse (Rubin & Wylie, 2009). Steps have been taken to convert prescription-only medicinal products commonly prescribed for the treatment of chronic conditions, to make them available over-the-counter as well as those that are considered "lifestyle medications," including sildenafil and other PDE5i. Sildenafil, and indeed other drugs in this class, while initially targeting older males, have seen the greatest uptick in use among younger males, where the fastest growing group of consumers were men aged 18−45 years, and such use carries with it the concern that the drug is being used, not merely to fulfill a medical need, but rather a recreational use (Morales, Campos, & Cruz, 2005). It also well documented that the use of drugs such as sildenafil is used to counteract the erectile dysfunction that accompanies use of amphetamines (Rubin & Wylie, 2009). Young men using drugs and sidestepping the etiology of a condition to apply a "quick-fix" is hardly new, but there is an ethical and moral obligation incumbent on all in society, to help those who are vulnerable from being preyed upon.

Bibliography

Abramson, E. L., Patel, V., Pfoh, E. R., & Kaushal, R. (2016). How physician perspectives on e-prescribing evolve over time. A case study following the transition between EHRs in an outpatient clinic. *Applasma Clinical Information, 7*(4), 994–1006. https://doi.org/10.4338/ACI-2016-04-RA-0069

Achar, S., Sinha, N., & Norcross, W. (2021). The adoption and increased use of electronic prescribing of controlled substances. *Journal of Medical Regulation, 107*(2), 8–16. https://doi.org/10.30770/2572-1852-107.2.8

Bates, C., Laciak, R., Southwick, A., & Bishoff, J. (2011). Overprescription of postoperative narcotics: A look at postoperative pain medication delivery, consumption and disposal in urological practice. *Journal of Urology, 185*(2), 551–555. https://doi.org/10.1016/j.juro.2010.09.088

Bell, J. (2010). The global diversion of pharmaceutical drugs: Opiate treatment and the diversion of pharmaceutical opiates: A clinician's perspective. *Addiction, 105*(9), 1531–1537. https://doi.org/10.1111/j.1360-0443.2010.03014.x

Brimley, S., Natale, C., Dick, B., Pastuszak, A., Khera, M., Baum, N., & Raheem, O. A. (2021). The emerging critical role of telemedicine in the urology clinic: A practical guide. *Sexual Medicine Reviews, 9*(2), 289–295. https://doi.org/10.1016/j.sxmr.2020.12.002

Gabrielsen, J. S., Najari, B. B., Alukal, J. P., & Eisenberg, M. L. (2016). Trends in testosterone prescription and public health concerns. *Urologic Clinics of North America, 43*(2), 261–271. https://doi.org/10.1016/j.ucl.2016.01.010

Grossman, J. M., Gerland, A., Reed, M. C., & Fahlman, C. (2007). Physicians' experiences using commercial e-prescribing systems. *Health Affairs (Millwood), 26*(3), w393–404. https://doi.org/10.1377/hlthaff.26.3.w393

Gu, Y., Liang, X., Wu, W., Liu, M., Song, S., Cheng, L., … Yao, K. (2009). Multicenter contraceptive efficacy trial of injectable testosterone undecanoate in Chinese men. *Journal of Clinical Endocrinology Metabolism, 94*(6), 1910–1915. https://doi.org/10.1210/jc.2008-1846

Hall, S. A., Link, C. L., Hu, J. C., Eggers, P. W., & McKinlay, J. B. (2009). Drug treatment of urological symptoms: Estimating the magnitude of unmet need in a community-based sample. *BJU International, 104*(11), 1680–1688. https://doi.org/10.1111/j.1464-410X.2009.08686.x

Kirana, P. S., Gudeloglu, A., Sansone, A., Fode, M., Reisman, Y., Corona, G., & Burri, A. (2020). E-sexual health: A position statement of the European Society for Sexual Medicine. *Journal of Sexual Medicine, 17*(7), 1246–1253. https://doi.org/10.1016/j.jsxm.2020.03.009

Lydia Feinstein, P., & Matlaga, Brian (2018). *Urologic diseases in America*. Washington DC: US Government Printing Office.

Malik, R. D., Wang, C. E., Lapin, B., Lakeman, J. C., & Helfand, B. T. (2015). Characteristics of men undergoing testosterone replacement therapy and adherence to follow-up recommendations in metropolitan multicenter health care system. *Urology, 85*(6), 1382–1388. https://doi.org/10.1016/j.urology.2015.01.027

Morales, K., Campos, T., & Cruz, A. R. (2005). Erectile dysfunction. *BMJ, 331*(Suppl. S6). https://doi.org/10.1136/sbmj.0512453

Nieschlag, E., Vorona, E., Wenk, M., Hemker, A. K., Kamischke, A., & Zitzmann, M. (2011). Hormonal male contraception in men with normal and subnormal semen parameters. *International Journal of Andrology, 34*(6 Pt 1), 556–567. https://doi.org/10.1111/j.1365-2605.2011.01142.x

Rubin, N., & Wylie, K. (2009). Should sildenafil be available over the counter? *British Medical Bulletin, 90*, 53−62. https://doi.org/10.1093/bmb/ldp001

Shahinyan, R. H., Amighi, A., Carey, A. N., Yoffe, D. A., Hodge, D. C., Pollard, M. E., … Eleswarapu, S. V. (2020). Direct-to-consumer internet prescription platforms overlook crucial pathology found during traditional office evaluation of young men with erectile dysfunction. *Urology, 143*, 165−172. https://doi.org/10.1016/j.urology.2020.03.067

Wood, D. (2015). Drug diversion. *Australian Prescriber, 38*(5), 164−166. https://doi.org/10.18773/austprescr.2015.058

Ziegelmann, M. J., Joseph, J. P., Glasgow, A. E., Tyson, M. D., Pak, R. W., Gazelka, H. M., … Gettman, M. T. (2019). Wide variation in opioid prescribing after urological surgery in tertiary care centers. *Mayo Clinical Proceedings, 94*(2), 262−274. https://doi.org/10.1016/j.mayocp.2018.08.035

Index

'Note: Page numbers followed by "f" indicate figures and "t" indicate tables.'